MILK MADNESS

WHY DRINKING MILK IS UDDERLY INSANE!

Gregory Cheadle
JD, MPA

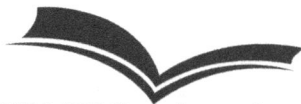

TEACH Services, Inc.
P U B L I S H I N G
www.TEACHServices.com • (800) 367-1844

Copyright © 2022 Gregory Cheadle
Copyright © 2022 TEACH Services, Inc.
ISBN-13: 978-1-4796-1542-1 (Paperback)
ISBN-13: 978-1-4796-1543-8 (ePub)
Library of Congress Control Number: 2022917206

The website references in this book have been shortened using a URL shortener and redirect service called 1ref.us, which TEACH Services manages. If you find that a reference no longer works, please contact us and let us know which one is not working so that we can correct it. Any personal website addresses that the author included are managed by the author. TEACH Services is not responsible for the accuracy or permanency of any links.

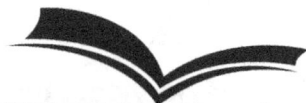

TEACH Services, Inc.
PUBLISHING
www.TEACHServices.com • (800) 367-1844

*This book is dedicated to those who are seeking
a much better life!*

CONTENTS

Chapter 1

CALCIUM AND OTHER UDDER NONSENSE

It is amazing that in this country with its wealth of intelligence, economic wealth, and education, a country with millions of college graduates, thousands upon thousands of attorneys and physicians, its citizens engage heartily in one of the most nonsensical acts imaginable, the drinking of cow's milk! It just goes to show that academic education is not enough to prevent people from doing nonsensical things when they have been indoctrinated for decades by the dairy industry.

Take a moment and try to be objective in your thinking. Would you agree with me that: 1) the milk from a human is designed for baby humans; 2) that milk from a cow is designed for a baby cow; 3) if a baby cow was given human milk that it would not get the same nourishment that it would get from the milk of a cow? If you answered all of the above questions with a simple "Yes," then why is it not strange that humans drink cow's milk? It should seem bizarre on three levels. First, it should seem bizarre that we would feed human babies the milk of a cow rather than the milk of a human. Secondly, it should seem bizarre that adult humans would be drinking milk at all. Thirdly, it should seem bizarre that adult humans would drink the milk of another species.

What exactly is milk? The white liquid that is often used for breakfast cereals is a smorgasbord of chemicals ranging from water to a plethora of hormones. Every drop of cow's milk contains any number of hormones. Specifically, cow's milk contains: pituitary hormones—Growth Hormone (GH), Thyroid Stimulating Hormone (TSH), Follicle Stimulating Hormone (FSH), Luteinizing Hormone (LH), Adrencorticotrpic Hormone (ACTH), PRL, and Oxytocin; Hypothalamic hormones:—Thyrotropin

7

Releasing Hormone (TRH), Luteinizing Hormone-Releasing Hormone (LHRH), Somatostatin, PRL inhibiting factor, PRL releasing factor, GnRH, GRH); steroid hormones:—Estradiol, Estriol, Progesterone, testosterone, ketosteroids, and corticosterone. Additionally, there are a host of other hormones from the pancreas, thyroid, parathyroid, adrenal glands, and gonads. In addition, there are prostaglandins and neuro and gastropeptides in milk. There is also a substance in milk known as IGF-1, which is short for Insulin Growth Factor 1.

Given the complexity of the chemical composition of milk, especially the number and concentration of hormones, it is clear that milk is actually a hormonal and chemical transport medium designed for growth and is more than just a beverage.

The milk of each species is designed to best suit the needs of its own growing infants. For instance, the amount of protein, calcium, fat, phosphorous, etc., in the milk of humans, cows, cats, and goats varies considerably. Human milk has all the nutrients in the proper amounts that a growing human baby needs. Cow's milk has all the nutrients in their proper amounts necessary for the growth and maturation of a calf. Obviously, the nutrient needs of both differ considerably.

The average newborn baby weighs about seven and a half pounds.[1] It takes about six months for the newborn to double its birth weight and about a year to triple it. A newborn calf weighs between fifty-seven and ninety-one pounds and will double its birth weight in only one and a half months.[2] It will weigh almost 1,000 pounds in a little over a year!!! Given the rate of weight increase, it is clear that the chemicals in human milk are in a form and concentration that makes them readily available for absorption and utilization in the system of the growing baby. The same holds true for the milk of a cow. Do you honestly think that the milk from a 1,000 to 1,500-pound cow with several stomachs is comparable to that found in a 130-pound human with only one stomach? It makes about as much sense for human babies to drink cow's milk as it does for calves to drink human milk. Perhaps now you can understand why your child cries and screams

---

1 Maressa Brown, "Your Newborn's Weight: Normal Gains and Losses and What the Average Baby Weighs," What to Expect, https://1ref.us/1wz (accessed May 25, 2022).
2 Linden, Bicalho, and Nydam, "Calf Birth Weight and It's association with Calf and Cow Survivability, Disease Incidence, Reproductive Performance, and Milk Production," *Journal of Dairy Science*, https://1ref.us/1x0 (accessed May 25, 2022).

when you give him/her a bottle of cow milk!!! Children are smarter than we think!!!

Milk is a Natural?

Milk is a Natural! was the slogan for another successful advertising campaign by the dairy industry. Yes, milk is a natural, BUT milk is a natural substance for the delivery of hormones for calves. However, we are not told the dirty side of the milk issue, that now more than ever, milk is a natural substance that causes disease in humans! Is it "natural" for humans to drink the milk of another species? Is there something about the human body that requires milk from another species? Even from the so-called "scientific" viewpoint of the philosophy of "evolution," it would seem that if humans required the milk of a cow, our "cousins," the chimps and monkeys, would be lining up behind every lactating cow they could find. Perhaps they are a lot smarter than we think!

The question then becomes—why are so many people drinking cow's milk? Tradition and habit and the ready availability are the main reasons why people in this country consume so much cow's milk. The reasons above are based on, and perpetuated by, the never-ceasing inculcating propaganda of the dairy industry. The dairy industry, like the meat industry, uses every form of media to make the general public neurotic about not getting enough calcium and that cow's milk will supply all of the calcium our bodies demand. Consequently, people are programmed to go out and buy milk, milk, and more milk to build strong bones!!! Just what the American Dairy Association wants them to do!

Education does have its dangers. There are some basic principles of psychology when employed properly, will cause a person to believe just about anything. One principle is if you tell someone something many times over an extended period of time, they will believe it. This was one of the tactics used by Hitler through one of his underlings, Joseph Goebbels. Another principle is that if someone in a position of "authority" says something, no matter how "strange" it sounds, it will likely be perceived as "truth" and will not be challenged. Another principle is that if there is an element of truth to the message, no matter how much falsehood is in the message, the message will be received as being "truth." Given the above, the most powerful persuasive technique would be to have someone in "authority" repeat the same message repeatedly for an extended period of time.

Let's look at a real-world problem and see how it is solved. The problem: getting humans to drink the milk of another species. The solution: set up a respectable authoritative body and have them spread the message that "humans need milk from a cow in order to have calcium, which is needed for strong teeth and bones."

Prior to 1970, milk promotion was done on the state and local level by contributions from milk producers. In 1970 the National Dairy Council and the American Dairy Association merged to form the United Dairy Industry Association.[3] In a move to increase the national promotion of milk, in 1983, congress enacted the Dairy and Tobacco Adjustment Act. Title I of this act authorized a national dairy promotion program (or, Check-off program) for generic dairy product promotion, research, and nutrition education. This self-help program is funded through a permanent 15¢/cwt. assessment on all milk production and is administered by a board of dairy farmers who are appointed by the Secretary of Agriculture. Shortly thereafter, the Secretary of Agriculture appointed the first board for the National Dairy Promotion and Research Board, at which point it started demand-building programs.

In 1995, board members of the National Dairy Promotion and Research Board and the National Dairy Industry Association created a new organization, Dairy Management Inc., which was responsible for increasing demand for U.S. dairy products.[4] Dairy Management Inc. then formed the U.S. Dairy Export Council.[5] Its role was to enhance the U.S. dairy industry's ability to serve international markets. Here we have an authority, a message that is spread repeatedly, and the message has an element of truth with which to cover its falsity. Nevertheless, this message has been ingrained in the minds of hundreds of millions of people throughout the world. The authoritative body is the National Dairy council. Its message they convey is simple—humans need milk from a cow in order to have sufficient calcium that is needed for strong teeth and bones. This message has been spread everywhere in this country for

---

3 "History," Undeniably Dairy, https://1ref.us/1x1 (accessed May 25, 2022).
4 "History," Undeniably Dairy, https://1ref.us/1x1 (accessed May 25, 2022).
5 "About Us," U.S. Dairy Export Council, https://1ref.us/1x2 (accessed May 25, 2022).

decades, and its influence is still hard to counter, despite overwhelming scientific evidence to the contrary.

The National Dairy Council supplied nutritional teaching aids to children in schools beginning as early as kindergarten with the propaganda that humans need milk from a cow in order to have calcium that is needed for strong teeth and bones. In addition, the National Dairy Council is bolstered by the UDSA since it is the job of the USDA to promote the consumption of agricultural products. The USDA, in the promotion of the food groups and pyramids over the years, was more concerned with the promotion of meat and dairy products than relying on science to determine the optimum food requirements of humans.

The National Dairy Council's message that milk is so important to the health of humans has been taken as gospel throughout the world unchallenged until recently.

Clearly, calcium is a very important element in the body. It makes up approximately 1.5 percent of our body mass and is necessary for bones and teeth.[6] It is needed for proper bone and cartilage formation and activation of hormones. Calcium must be in its ionic form in order to be used in blood clotting, muscle contraction, and for the conduction of nerve impulses. Calcium also neutralizes acid. It is interesting to note that dairy products are acid-forming because of the high amount of protein in milk. Therefore, as the amount of dairy products consumed increases, the amount of acid formed increases. The more acid that is formed, the more calcium that will be used to neutralize the acid; thus, a vicious cycle begins. This calls into question the validity of the RDA for calcium. Would not the amount of calcium needed be lower in people who do not consume dairy products?

Marketing–How to Make Junk Valuable

Safe, wholesome, and nutritious! That is what the dairy industry wants you to believe about milk, a substance that is safe, wholesome, and nutritious for calves but unsafe, unwholesome, and unfit for human consumption. In order to fool the public, the dairy industry spends millions of dollars each year on marketing, knowing that if you hear

---

6 Michael Schirber, "The Chemistry of Life: The Human Body," Live Science, https://1ref.us/1x3 (accessed May 25, 2022).

a lie long enough, you will eventually come to the point that it will be accepted as truth. The goal of the dairy industry is to blanket the world with misinformation to make dairy products an integral part of the daily American diet. The purpose of all of this is to make children lifelong consumers of dairy products. Unlike other species that become weaned from milk, the goal of the dairy industry is to make children lifelong consumers of milk, and they are working overtime to make their dream a reality.

The dairy industry has a multipronged attack plan in place to achieve its goal of making people lifelong dairy consumers. Under the guise of promoting health, the Child Nutrition and Fitness Initiative was developed to encourage good nutrition. Not surprisingly, dairy products were included in this plan that is targeted at the nation's schools. Moreover, the dairy industry is busy promoting "Healthy Behaviors," such as choosing low-fat and non-fat dairy products encouraged by the Dietary Guideline for Americans. In order to make their position appear valid and to be proactive in promoting junk science as real science behind their data, the National Dairy Council aggressively targets public health officials and leaders with their propaganda.

In 2003, the 3-A-Day dairy program was launched. Its purpose was to increase the average daily consumption of dairy products from 1.6 servings to 3, under the guise of addressing the nation's calcium crises, which, ironically, dairy products are responsible for in a large measure. This strategy has even hit the presses of the mainstream media. The March 20, 2009, issue of U.S. News & World Report has what appears to be an article written by Kerry Hannon about the benefits of milk. The article talks about five things you should know about your kids and milk. In the article Kerry says that children need to drink more milk because it contains "essential nutrients and vitamins …" Not surprisingly, Kerry listed the vitamins but conveniently failed to list the "essential nutrients." As such, it makes one wonder how essential the essential nutrients really are.

Another part of the strategy is to make dairy products available around the clock in whatever form and wherever the consumer desires. This is being done by the building of partnerships with various corporations such as Starbucks, McDonald's, Subway, Wendy's, Burger King, Sonic Drive-In, many of which now have chocolate and white milk in single-serve plastic bottles in over 60,000 restaurants in the country. Sonic Drive-In began offering string cheese on its kids' menu. Subway got into the act by offering a low-fat yogurt with its "Fresh Fit for Kids" promotion, thanks to market research provided by the dairy Checkoff program.

Another target of the dairy industry is the exportation of dairy products. The volume and value of exports of dairy products have increased nearly more than four-fold from 2005 to 2015.[7] U.S. dairy products have been introduced via in-store promotions and consumer "education." Additionally, U.S. dairy suppliers formed alliances with Mexican restaurant chains for them to use cheese in their menu items. In Japan, thanks to the efforts of the dairy industry, exports of dairy products increased 30 percent in one year alone.

In addition to promoting dairy products on the consumer level, the dairy industry has also as its focus the inclusion of dairy products, namely, cheese, whey, and milk powder, as ingredients in a wide range of products.

In order to keep attacks against its junk science, propaganda, and false claims from being explored, discovered, and brought to light, the dairy Check-off program is on the watch twenty-four hours a day, seven days a week to put a "spin" on any issue that arises in the media or elsewhere that could endanger their profits. They have staff available to counter activists, negative media reports, and any opposition that may arise. Quoting from Check-off's own materials (www.dairycheckoff.com), you can see that they mean business:

"Working with the National Milk Producers Federation, U.S. Dairy Export Council®, International Dairy Foods Association, and Milk Processor Education Program, the dairy checkoff maintains a comprehensive issues management network. When special-interest groups oppose dairy's role in a healthy diet, checkoff staff educates the media and other thought leaders about the sound science that supports dairy's health benefits and the responsible production practices that ensure milk quality and safety. Dairy producers and allied industry representatives participate in Check-off-funded communications training that prepares them to educate the media and public about the realities of modern dairy production."

After 1970, the amount of milk consumed per capita began to decrease. In 1980, the per capita consumption of beverage milks was 234 pounds. In 1990, the per capita consumption of beverage milks was 220

---

7 Market Information—Top Charts, U.S. Dairy Export Council, https://1ref.us/1x4 (accessed May 25, 2022).

pounds. By 2000, the per capita consumption of milk decreased to 197 pounds. In order to increase consumption of milk, the dairy industry had to boost the image of milk to make it more appealing, accent its alleged value, and make it appear to be an essential dietary component. Hence, the media blitz of ad campaigns and propaganda – "Milk is a natural!" "Milk does a body good!" and the now-famous, "Got Milk?" In addition, the dairy industry began to increase the popularity of dairy products via marketing and availability of products. This strategy has proven to be effective. In 1994, the average person in the U.S. consumed 579 pounds of dairy products. By 2020, the average amount of dairy products a person consumed in the U.S. had risen to 655 pounds.[8]

Got Milk?

Milk production is a big business and a very political one at that. Undoubtedly, it is due to politics that there is so much milk around. In 1980, 128,400,000,000 pounds of milk were produced in this country. In addition, we imported an additional 2,100,000,000 pounds! In order to achieve this amount of milk production from the 128,406,000 dairy cows, the average dairy cow produced 11,900 pounds of milk! A decade later, in 1990, the amount of milk produced in this country climbed to 147,700,000,000 pounds from 147,721,000 dairy cattle, with the average cow producing 14,782 pounds (about twice the weight of an elephant) of milk, nearly 3000 more pounds than a decade earlier![9] Furthermore, we imported 2,500,000,000 pounds that year! By 2019, milk production had climbed to 218,000,000,000 pounds! The average amount of milk produced per cow (based on an average of 9,336,000 dairy cows on farms) climbed to 23,391 pounds (about the weight of a school bus)![10] No matter how you figure it, that is a whole lot of milk!!!

In 2019, the state of Alabama had the distinction of having the least productive cows because their cows' average production of milk is only 12,000 pounds. The great state of Michigan, of all places, has the distinction of having the most productive cows, with each cow averaging

8 Dairy Data, USDA Economic Research Service, https://1ref.us/1x5 (accessed May 25, 2022). See Data Set for Dairy products: Per capita consumption, United States (Annual).
9 Don P. Blayney, "The Changing Landscape of U.S. Milk Production," USDA Statistical Bulletin Number 978 (June 2002): 2, https://1ref.us/1x6 (accessed https://1ref.us/1x6).
10 Blayney, "The Changing Landscape," 7.

26,725 pounds of milk, more than double the milk production of cows in Alabama.[11] Also, in 2019, the state of Rhode Island had the lowest number

> *California had the highest number of dairy cattle*

of dairy cattle, 700, and the lowest amount of milk produced of the 50 states, 10,600,000 pounds. California had the highest number of dairy cattle, 1,734,000, and the highest amount of milk produced, 40,564,000,000 pounds.[12] The total milk produced was 217,500,000,000 pounds in 2019.[13]

Is all of the milk produced each year consumed by citizens of the United States? No! Millions of pounds of dry milk, cheese, and butter are stored by the government every year. The amount of money the government spends each year to purchase, transport, and store the dry milk, butter, and cheese is nothing more than a collateral expense of paying billions in dairy and farm subsidies. This is one of the most wasteful and nonsensical welfare programs in existence.

Before milk became such a "necessity," dairy cows were milked by hand, free to roam around the farm and graze in a natural manner. Perhaps that's why in 1945, the average cow produced only 4,600 pounds of milk. Today milk has gone hi-tech, and the cow's genetic makeup has been and continues to be, exploited. There are sperm banks for cows for high milk yield and high milk fat content. There are even surrogate cows! The latest "advance" is milk from cloned cows, with the goal in sight to have a cow produce 40,000 pounds (about twice the weight of a school bus) of milk per year!!! Talk about "Got milk"! This can be attributed to the big business mentality of agribusiness.

The family-owned and run farms are being taken over by large corporation entities. In 1970, the number of farms with dairy cows was 648,000, but by 2006 the number had fallen to 75,000. The total number of dairy cows increased as well during this period, from 12 million in 1970 to 9.1 million in 2006. The average herd size increased from 19 cows per farm in 1970 to 120 cows by 2006. Though the number of dairy farms decreased as well as the number of dairy cows, surprisingly, the amount of

---

11 "Milk Production—February 2020," USDA National Agricultural Statistics Service, https://1ref.us/1x7 (accessed May 25, 2022), 8.
12 "Milk Production—February 2020," 8.
13 M. Shahbandeh, "Total Milk Production In the United States from 1999–2022 (In Million Pounds)," Statista, https://1ref.us/1x8 (accessed May 25, 2022).

milk produced increased. This increase was due to a doubling of the milk produced per cow.[14]

There are dairy farms with more than 15,000 cows, but the most common dairy farms have between 1,000–5,000 cows. The smallest dairy farms, those with thirty or fewer cows, made up 30 percent of all dairy farms but only accounted for 1 percent of milk produced.[15] As of 2019 there were only 37,468 licensed dairy farms in the U.S.[16] With the increase in large corporations taking over the food supply, the small farmer is disadvantaged and simply cannot compete in the marketplace.

Milking the Public ... Welfare for Farmers!

When it comes to welfare, there is usually a negative connotation that goes along with it. However, when it comes to the dairy industry, government welfare in the form of subsidies and price supports, payment for losses, etc., is not seen as welfare by the sacred dairy industry! The dairy industry is one of the most powerful and guarded industries in Washington. Unfortunately, those who lobby for the dairy industry tend to ignore the smaller farmers and instead work to bolster the coffers of the mammoth factory dairies with all manner of tax breaks and benefits to quash the small farmer and monopolize the market. This also has the effect of forcing the small farmer out of business and allowing the larger farmers to scoop up farms at bargain prices. There is an old adage, "the rich get richer, and the poor get poorer." I don't have anything against the "rich" per se. However, I do take issue when wealth is obtained via complicity and duplicity, especially when the arm of government is employed to achieve their goals.

One dirty secret about the dairy industry is that it is subsidized heavily to offset the increasingly low demand. In 2018, 42 percent of the revenue for dairy farmers in the U.S. came from some form of government program. Some accounts have the figure as high as 70+ percent. In other words, the dairy farmers cannot look down on those receiving welfare because many

---

14 "Changes In the Size and Location of U.S. Dairy Farms," USDA, https://1ref.us/1x9 (accessed May 25, 2022).
15 "Changes In the Size and Location of U.S. Dairy Farms."
16 Jim Dickrell, "More Than 2,700 U.S. Dairy Farms Closed In 2018," Dairy Herd Management, https://1ref.us/1xa (accessed May 25, 2022).

of them would not have anything if it were not for the government welfare that they receive. The Agricultural Act of 2014 was to bring about reforms in the commodity and crop insurance programs. The reforms took on the form of less transparency and more money in subsidies. In 2015, $24.7 billion was paid in direct and indirect subsidies. In 2016, the amount of money for subsidies increased by more than 70 percent to $43 billion. In 2018, the amount decreased to $36.3 billion, which was nearly 50 percent more than what was spent in 2015.[17]

It is no accident that the highest-ranking members of government are also involved with some of the largest private businesses, investment banks, and law firms in the nation. A sad commentary on our society is the simple fact that if you want to make a lot of money, all you have to do is have government step in to make your product or service mandatory. Better yet, have the government subsidize your product or service because it is something that you've convinced them is for the better good of society.

The general public looks with gross disdain upon those members of society who manage to subsist on welfare, or more properly called today, public assistance. Moreover, those who are on some form of public assistance are often ashamed of so being. Interestingly, there are other forms of welfare, the recipients of which do not hold their heads down in shame, i.e., those involved in the military industrial complex, the criminal justice industrial complex, farmers, etc. I will only touch on the latter here, as the former are the material for several books alone.

Unlike many other businesses, the U.S. government steps in to help dairy farmers make ends meet. They do so by providing subsidies and making the price. Subsidies are nothing more than a form of welfare. This is one form of welfare that is rarely discussed in the media. Generally, when welfare is discussed in the media, particularly in print and visual media, the story tends to revolve around a black female with children or other woman of color. However, the dairy welfare beneficiaries tend to be white males of varying income levels. One would think that the poor family dairy farm with just a few dozen or so dairy cows is the type that would receive the subsidy. Strangely enough, the poor family dairy farmer,

---

17 Stephanie Luiz, "My Beef with Dairy: How the US Government Is Bailing Out a Dying Industry," Northeastern University Political Review, https://1ref.us/1xb (accessed May 25, 2022).

who really could use a helping hand, gets a pocketful of change compared to the millions of dollars the rich dairy farm owners receive. (See Table 1)

Consider, for instance, the Gallo family, yes, of the famous winemaker family. A member of the famous winemaking family owned at one time one of the largest dairy herds in the nation numbering 22,000 head, range-residing on more than 10,000 acres (about half the area of Cleveland, Ohio) of California land![18] The family currently owns one of the largest cheese-processing facilities in California, which alone grosses tens of millions of dollars a year! You would think that with all of the land, cattle, and cheese that he produces that he would not be in need of any government assistance. The Gallo cattle company has raked in at least $2,058,154 in farm subsidies from 1995 – 2020 for raising crops to feed their cattle. This is in addition to the $1,549,024 received during the same period for dairy subsidies for making milk that no one needs.[19] This is in stark contrast to the approximately $36,000 average payment most dairy farmers received that year.

Chuck Ahlem, the former undersecretary of the California Department of Food and Agriculture, is the founder of the largest single-site cheese factory in the world. It processes more than 12,500,000 pounds (5,5000,000 liters) of milk received from more than 200 dairies and 160,000 cows each day. This staggering amount of milk is what is needed for the 1,300,000 pounds (591 plus metric tons) of cheese the plant produces each day.

One would think that with such vast wealth as Ahlem has, he would not be in need of government help. Through the years, Ahlem and his family have received hundreds of thousands of dollars from the government in the form of subsidies.[20] He received subsidies for his dairy and livestock operations as well as to grow corn and wheat that he fed to his own cattle!!!!

Unfortunately for the American taxpayer, the Gallo and the Ahlem family look like true welfare recipients compared to a number of other farmers. The owner(s) of the McNutt Brothers Dairy in Dublin, Texas, had a wonderful year in 2002 at the expense of the American taxpayer.

---

18 James Carper, "Joseph Gallo Farms Is California's 'Green' Cheesemaker," Dairyfoods.com, https://1ref.us/1xc (accessed May 25, 2022); "USDA Subsidy Information for Gallo Cattle Company Lp," EWG, https://1ref.us/1xd (accessed May 25, 2022).
19 "Dairy Program Subsidies In California, 1995–2020," EWG, https://1ref.us/1xe (accessed May 25, 2022).
20 "EWG Farm Subsidy Database," EWG, https://1ref.us/1xf (accessed May 25, 2022).

In 2002, the McNutt Brothers Dairy received nearly $13,500,000 in dairy subsidies![21]

The top 1 percent of farmers (15,443) receiving crop subsidies average more than $125,000 per year from Uncle Sam! Furthermore, the top 1 percent receive 17 percent of the total amount of crop subsidies! The top 20 percent (308,864) of those receiving crop subsidies hoard 84 percent of the crop subsidies and had an average annual amount of $31,494. The remaining 80percent (1,235,460) of the farmers receiving crop subsidies received a paltry average annual amount of only $1,503!!!

If you really want to make a living as a farmer at the expense of the government, then perhaps you should consider having a farm in the district of one of the members of the House Agricultural Committee. In 2017, thirty-three members of congress and their immediate family members took in more than $15,000,000 in farm subsidies between 1995 and 2016. Many of these members of congress grow crops that make them eligible for crop insurance subsidies as well, but conveniently, these subsidies cannot be disclosed to the public![22]

Table 1 Top Dairy Subsidy Recipients 1995 to 2020[23]

Rank	Recipient	Location	Subsidy
1	McNutt Bros Dairy	Dublin, TX	$13,637,653
2	Zonneveld Dairies	Laton, CA	$1,710,000
3	Gallo Cattle Co.	Atwater, CA	$1,549,024
4	Hein Hettinga	Ontario, CA	$1,287,115
5	Las Uvas Valley	Hatch, NM	$1,279,539
6	Nickerson Brothers	Zolfo Springs, FL	$1,272,614
7	Larson Dairy Inc	Okeechobee, FL	$1,265,812
8	McArthur Farms	Okeechobee, FL	$1,244,351
9	Aardema Dairy	Wendell, ID	$1,173,541

21 "USDA Subsidy Information for Mcnutt Bros Dairy," EWG, https://1ref.us/1xg (accessed May 25, 2022).
22 Jared Hayes, "Federal Lawmakers Harvest $15 Million In Farm Subsidies," EWG, https://1ref.us/1xh (accessed May 25, 2022).
23 "Dairy Program Subsidies In the United States, 1995–2020," EWG, https://1ref.us/1xi (accessed May 25, 2022).

Rank	Recipient	Location	Subsidy
10	Big Sky Dairy	Jerome, ID	$1,1655,872
11	Alvin Souza Dairy	Tulare CA	$1,055,895
12	Warren Hettinga	Tipton, CA	$1,052,864
13	Foster Farms	Hickman, CA	$1,012,140
14	Dores Dairy Ptn	Stevinson, CA	$968,505
15	Bosman Dairy	Tipton, CA	$925,689
16	Lemstra Dairy	Tulare, CA	$910,008
17	Vander Schaaf	Escalon, CA	$856,481
18	Cheyenne Dairy	Dexter, NM	$841,266
19	Joe Soares Dairy	Delhi CA	$833,261
20	Carlos Echeverria	Bakersfield, CA	$829,639

* USDA data are not "transparent" for many payments made to recipients through most cooperatives. Recipients of payments made through most cooperatives, and the amounts, have not been made public.

** Data for 2019 is incomplete, it only includes Market Facilitation Program payments between January1, 2019 and October 31, 2019

More Milk?

As if the cows are not busy enough producing voluminous amounts of milk that they currently produce, there is a trend to make these cows produce even more milk, up to 20 percent more, by giving them rBGH, a synthetic hormone.

After one of the biggest cover-ups, scandals, corporate power grabs, and manipulations in the history of the FDA, a synthetic hormone called rBGH (recombinant bovine growth hormone) was approved by federal officials for use in milk cows in the U.S. When the U.S. Food and Drug Administration (FDA) declared rBGH "safe" for use in milk cows, Monsanto, the chemical company, began selling its version of the drug to dairy farmers. Other companies eyeing the business are Eli Lilly, Upjohn, and American Cyanamid. Monsanto's version of the drug is intended to be injected into milk cows every two weeks to stimulate milk production by 5 percent to 20 percent. Consumer and farm organizations, including Consumers Union, have presented evidence that byproducts of this hormone treatment are measurable in milk and are not safe for humans or for cows. The organizations also say approval of rBGH clearly violated FDA's own regulations. The organizations want the product withdrawn from the market, and they want hormone-containing milk labeled so consumers can make an informed choice about the milk they buy. Conventional rBGH-free brands are typically labeled "rBGH-free," "rBST-free" or "no artificial hormones."[24]

A handful of farm and consumer organizations have been waging a war against a coalition of agrichemical companies backed by top officials of the U.S. Food and Drug Administration (FDA) and the U.S. Department of Agriculture (USDA). At the heart of the war is the question of the safety of milk and the right of consumers to know what chemicals and drugs have been added to the milk they buy. Consumer advocates say the public has a right to know. The agrichemical industry, the FDA, and the USDA say that the right to know is not a right!

American consumers unquestionably do not want milk that contains genetically engineered hormones, and that they want milk labeled so they can make an informed choice in the grocery store. In response to consumer concerns, the FDA and Monsanto have turned a deaf ear. The FDA has even gone as far as to warn grocery stores not to label milk as free of the hormone. Monsanto, in a move to quell a rebellion, sued two milk processors that labeled milk as free of the hormone.

It is not by chance coincidence that the FDA and Monsanto are speaking in concert on this issue. The FDA official responsible for the agency's labeling policy, Michael R. Taylor, is a former partner of King & Spaulding, a Washington, D.C., law firm. King & Spaulding brought lawsuits on behalf of Monsanto. Taylor, a lawyer, is a classic product of the "revolving door." Starting in 1980, Taylor worked for the FDA for four years as executive assistant to the commissioner. In 1984 Taylor joined King & Spaulding and remained there until 1991; during that time,

> *Would it be so hard to find honest dairy people who are not using rBGH to produce their milk?*

the law firm represented Monsanto while the company was seeking FDA approval of rBGH. In 1991, President Bush's FDA Commissioner, David A. Kessler, Jr., revolved Taylor back into FDA as assistant commissioner for policy. Kessler himself was retained by President Clinton, as was Taylor. It was Taylor who signed the FEDERAL REGISTER notice

---

24 "Know Your Milk: Does It Have Artificial Hormones?" Physicians for Social Responsibility (PSR), Oregon Chapter, https://1ref.us/1xj (accessed May 25, 2022).

warning grocery stores not to label milk as free of rBGH. By so doing, this gave Monsanto a powerful boost in its fight to prevent consumers from knowing whether or not their milk came from cows given rBGH. Rather than being concerned about the welfare of the general public, the FDA, in this case, is acting more like a guardian of corporate billions by offering two justifications for preventing labeling. Their first justification is that the FDA is not requiring anyone to keep track of who is using rBGH and who is not. In their minds, without a paper trail, grocery stores might make false claims if they said their milk was rBGH-free. Would it be so hard to find honest dairy people who are not using rBGH to produce their milk? The second lame justification that the FDA used was that there is virtually no difference between milk from cows injected with rBGH and cows not injected. Former FDA Commissioner Kessler has consistently opposed giving consumers a choice by labeling milk. He has said, "The public can be confident that milk and meat from BST-treated cows is safe to consume." (BST is Monsanto's name for rBGH.) And "There is virtually no difference in milk from treated and untreated cows."[25] Please be aware that the term "virtually" does not mean absolutely. It means almost! In other words, the FDA has been trying to dupe the public into thinking that there is "no" difference in the milk from cows given rBGH and cows not given rBGH. The truth is there is a difference between the milks. Fortunately, a considerable body of scientific evidence from around the world indicates that Commissioner Kessler was conveniently "stretching" the truth. Evidence indicates that milk from rBGH-treated cows is highly likely to contain more pus from infected cows' udders; more antibiotics given to cows to treat udder infections; an "off" taste and shortened shelf life because of the pus; higher fat content, and lower protein content; and more of a tumor-promoting chemical called IGF-I, which has been implicated in cancers of the colon, smooth muscle, and breast.

In return for accepting increased pus, more antibiotics, and a tumor-promoting chemical in their glass of milk, what benefits will consumers get? None, zero, nada, ziro, nunca! Even FDA says there are no consumer benefits. In fact, because the U.S. already produces a surplus of milk, which is purchased by Uncle Sam, increasing milk production with rBGH

---

25 Associated Press, "FDA Approves Milk-Boosting Drug for Cows," *L.A. Times Archives*, Nov. 7, 1993, https://1ref.us/1xk (accessed May 25, 2022).

will COST the taxpayer an additional $200 million or more each year, estimates Consumers Union.

The FDA's first justification could have easily been met by simply requiring Monsanto to maintain a public list of people, businesses, farms, etc., that buy rBGH or the farmers who use rBGH could be required to state that their milk is derived from cows given rBGH. This would afford grocery stores and milk wholesalers the opportunity to easily determine whether a given farmer is or is not using the rBGH. Would Monsanto ever voluntarily maintain a list of purchasers of its products? Not likely. Evidently, and with good reason, Monsanto fears that informed consumers might choose not to buy milk produced by rBGH-treated cows. In order to keep the money flowing into its corporate coffers, once again, the government has been tapped to be the pit bull to protect corporate profits while biting the derriere of the consumer.

Monsanto is taking desperate steps because it is desperate. Having spent approximately $300 million to develop rBGH, there is no way Monsanto would just relax and be a "good boy." Monsanto has taken a bath financially in recent times. It has been sued and had terrible publicity over several chemicals that it insisted were safe. The herbicide 2,4,5-T used in Agent Orange in Vietnam, and PCBs, which Congress banned in 1976, are just a couple of examples.

For nearly sixty years, U.S. dairy farmers have been producing more milk than Americans consume. In order to keep the dairy industry from going bankrupt because of the forces of supply and demand, the government purchases surplus milk. This "price support" program is nothing more than another form of welfare for dairy farmers under the guise of assuring the future of the nation's milk supply. Billions of dollars are paid to dairy farmers each year by the government to purchase surplus milk. The problem was so out of control that about twenty years ago, Congress passed the Food Security Act in an attempt to reduce the total cost of the dairy price support program by reducing the number of dairy herds. The government paid farmers to kill their cows and stop dairy farming for five years. Approximately 14,000 farmers signed up for this voluntary program. The program was responsible for slaughtering 1.55 million milk cows. However, what many other farmers simply did was increase the number of dairy cows in their herds! This led again to excessive milk production.

Where does the excess milk that the government purchases from dairy farmers go? In 2016 the excess amount of milk that was produced was so large that dairy farmers dumped more than forty-three million gallons of it in the ground. They literally threw it away all in a dying effort to keep the price of an ever-growing unwanted substance afloat![26] Excess milk also goes back to the farmers to feed their cows!!! Over one billion pounds of skim milk is turned into powder and stored by our government every year. This excess milk is also turned into cheese. In 2019, there were 1.4 BILLION pounds of government cheese in storage.[27] The rental fee to store all of this useless and wasteful substance amounts to tens of millions of dollars each year. We give the dairy farmers billions of dollars in subsidies and price support for a substance that is worthless. We spend millions more to store it. That which we do not store we give back to the dairy farmers to feed their cows to make more milk to purchase and store and feed back to them. Hmmm … If this is not welfare, I don't know what is!

Let me make certain you understand how our government works. The FDA allows a hormone on the market that will allow dairy cows to produce up to 20 percent more milk, despite evidence of health risks to the general population and the dairy cows. The government makes it almost a criminal act for farmers to label the milk from their non-rBGH cows as free from the Monsanto drug. Excessive milk production leads to lower prices paid to dairy farmers. The lower prices mean more subsidies paid to farmers. The excessive milk produced is more than the U.S. population can stomach, and the rest of the world refuses to stomach it. Consequently, we are forced to turn it into powder and store it underground and pay storage fees in excess of millions of dollars per year. The good news is that in some cases, the milk powder is fed back to dairy cattle to produce even more milk on a not-so-rainy day!!! Hmmm …

Many are no doubt aware that calcium as a nutrient is responsible for the formation and metabolism of bone. Nearly all of the calcium in the body is in the form of calcium hydroxyapatite ($Ca10[PO4]6[OH]2$). However, calcium is also found in the bloodstream throughout the body,

---

26 Kelsey Gee, "America's Dairy Farmers Dump 43 Million Gallons of Excess Milk," *The Wall Street Journal,* https://1ref.us/1xl (accessed May 25, 2022).

27 Gene Baur, "The Best Way to Help Dairy Farmers Is to Get Them Out of Dairy Farming," *The Washington Post,* https://1ref.us/1xm (accessed May 25, 2022).

which makes calcium readily available to meet the needs of muscles, nerves, blood vessels, and a host of other functions. Contrary to popular belief, bones are not stagnant or fixed, but they are in a constant state of being broken down, repaired, and remodeled as the body's need for calcium requires. This process is largely regulated by the parathyroid hormone and its interplay with vitamin D. Hence, bones serve as the depository for calcium.

Calcium from dairy products such as milk, cheese, and yogurt, is touted so much by the dairy industry that it could readily lead one to believe that such products are the only ideal source of calcium for humans. As a matter of fact, the dairy industry has done such an excellent job of promoting dairy products that 60–72 percent of dietary calcium in the United States comes from dairy products. The minor sources of calcium come from vegetables (7 percent); grains (5 percent); legumes (4 percent); fruit (3 percent); meat, poultry, and fish (3 percent); eggs (2 percent); and miscellaneous foods (3 percent). In Asian countries that are not in the cross-hairs of the propaganda of the dairy industry, calcium from dairy products makes up only 20–23 percent of the total intake.[28]

What is not discussed or made known to the general public is the amount of calcium that is absorbed by the body, as well as the calcium that is lost when one consumes large amounts of animal protein in the form of dairy products and meat. In general, the bioavailability or the amount of calcium that can be absorbed from a given substance is 30 percent from milk and even less from cheese. Though we are told that milk contains a lot of calcium, the reality is that though a cup of milk may have 300 mg of calcium, only 100 mg of it is likely to be absorbed. However, the bioavailability of calcium from some vegetables such as bok choy, broccoli, and kale is nearly double that of dairy products.[29] Kale, as well as broccoli, are rich in calcium and low in oxalate. This explains the high absorption rate of calcium of 40.9 percent, which is even higher than in milk (32.1 percent). As plants increase in oxalate, there is a decrease in their calcium absorption rate.[30] Products made from whole grains such as rye bread have

28 Fujita T. Osteoporosis-east and west. *Calcif Tiss Int* 48 (1991): 151–152.
29 A Ross, C Taylor, A. Yaktine, H. Del Valle, "Dietary Reference Intakes for Calcium and Vitamin D," *Institute of Medicine (US) Committee to Review Dietary Reference Intakes for Vitamin D and Calcium* (2011), https://1ref.us/1y7 (accessed June 2, 2022).
30 R. Heaney, C Weaver, R. Recker, "Calcium Absorbability from Spinach," *The American Journal of Clinical Nutrition* 47, no. 4 (April 1988): 707–709.

significant amounts of calcium with 107 mg (73 mg per 100 g). One cup of dried uncooked figs has the same amount of calcium as one cup of milk, 300 mg. Nuts are also a good source of dietary calcium. Sesame seeds are an exceptional source of plant-based calcium with about 280 mg per oz. The second most important source of calcium among Mexican Americans is corn tortillas.[31]

The amount of calcium that is excreted in the urine is directly correlated with the level of dietary protein intake. In a 95-day metabolic study, diets supplying 12 g nitrogen or 36 g nitrogen and approximately 1,400 mg calcium per day were compared for the amount of calcium that was excreted in the urine. The amount of calcium increased rapidly and significantly from an average of 191 mg/day on the 12 g nitrogen diet to 277 mg/day on the 36 g nitrogen diet. The apparent absorption of calcium was relatively the same calcium, so that overall calcium balance was − 37 mg/day on the 12 g nitrogen diet and significantly lower at − 137 mg/day in those who consumed the high protein diet. Levels of urinary hydroxyproline, serum insulin, and parathyroid hormone were not significantly increased by high intakes of protein. The most likely reason for the increase in calcium in the urine was a decrease in the fractional reabsorption of calcium by the kidneys. Given these results, the consumption of high calcium diets is unlikely to prevent the negative calcium balance and probable bone loss induced by the consumption of high protein diets. Even when consuming upwards of 1,400 mg of CA per day, one can lose up to 4 percent of their bone mass each day when consuming a high protein diet.[32] Additionally, milk is low in boron and high in phosphorous and protein, all of which lead to calcium loss.

In summary, high intake of animal protein leads to increased calcium in the urine, which will be excreted. High intake of sodium also leads to increased calcium in the urine which will be excreted. Hence, a diet rich in meat and dairy will lead to increased calcium excretion. Again, though you may take in dairy products because they are high in calcium, you will only absorb a fraction of the calcium present, AND you will lose calcium due to high animal protein consumption.

---

31 "DRI: Dietary Reference Intakes," In *The Essential Guide to Nutrient Requirements* (Washington: The National Academies Press, 1997).

32 *American Journal of Clinical Nutrition* 32, no. 4 (1979): 741–749.

Chapter 2

SICK COWS, BAD MILK!

The marketing plans of the dairy industry have led multitudes to believe that dairy cows are healthy, happy creatures roaming freely on the farm and eating grass at their leisure. Tragically, the exact opposite is the plight of the average dairy cow. Today, the average dairy cow is a milk machine, not a cute "Happy cow," but an animal exploited, abused, and manipulated for just one thing, its milk. When a dairy cow can no longer produce milk in sufficient quantities that it becomes a liability rather than an asset, it will be sent speedily to slaughter while it can still stand up. Over its short lifespan, the rigors of being a dairy cow lend themselves to bone, muscle, joint, and nerve damage. The damage is often so severe that it results in the cow being unable to stand on its own, a condition known in the industry as lameness or milk fever. When a cow can no longer stand on its own, it is called a downer cow and worthless to the farmer and must be disposed of. Since 2004, the USDA has required that cattle are able to walk to slaughter after being inspected by a USDA veterinarian. This safety precaution was put in place largely to avert and minimize exposure to prions in cattle with Mad Cow disease. Consequently, such cattle are not allowed to be slaughtered and be placed in the U.S. food supply but will likely end up being rendered for animal food.

Bovine Coronaviruses

Bovine coronaviruses (BCoVs) cause respiratory and gastrointestinal infections in cattle. BCoV is a pneumoenteric virus that infects the upper and lower respiratory tract and intestine. This virus is shed in feces and nasal secretions and also infects the lung. BCoV is the cause of three distinct clinical syndromes in cattle: (1) calf diarrhea, (2) winter dysentery with hemorrhagic diarrhea in adults, and (3) respiratory infections in cattle of various ages, including the bovine respiratory disease complex or shipping fever of feedlot cattle.[33]

Downer Cattle—Help! Mooooo… "I've fallen down, and I can't get up!"

As stated earlier, a downer cow is a cow that is unable to stand. The reasons why cows become "Downers" range from exhaustion, broken bones, milk fever (hypocalcemia), mastitis, to Mad Cow disease. Another cause that seems to go unnoticed is the fact that dairy cows today are producing upwards of twenty times the amount of milk they produced naturally in 1900. Given that milk is rich in calcium, and a cow can only take in so much calcium, the remaining calcium comes from the bones! Little wonder that used up, exploited cows, break legs and cannot stand and become "Downers."

It should also be noted that the trip to the slaughterhouse is also exhausting for these already worn-out animals. By the time they reach the slaughterhouse, many of them are so tired that they just lay down and cannot get back up.

Somatic (Pus) Cells

Animals are the victims of a multitude of diseases. Animals can acquire diseases from the food they consume, by being exposed to other animals, and by viruses and bacteria. A large number of the dairy cows whose milk is consumed are literally sick, but also many of the diseases that they suffer from can be transmitted to humans!!!

Given the incessant push for cows to produce more and more milk, cows are now producing more milk than a calf could ever consume and far greater quantities than their udders were designed to produce and to accommodate. Decades ago, a commercial dairy cow would produce 4000 pounds of milk per year. Today there are dairy cows that produce over 77,000 pounds (the weight of more than seven elephants!) of milk per year!1 Additionally, having a machine remove milk from the udder is

33 Linda J. Saif, "Bovine Respiratory Coronavirus," *The Veterinary Clinics of North America, Food Animal Practice* 26, no. 2, 349–364, https://1ref.us/1xn (accessed June 1, 2022).

an unnatural process that takes its toll on the udder. However, this comes with a cost because you can only push nature so far. One of the results of this unnatural stress on the udder is an increased risk of infections in and on the udder of the cow. To fight this increased risk for infections, somatic cells (SC) are released into the milk to fight infection and for tissue repair.

There are two types of bacteria or pathogens (contagious and environmental) that can be found in the udders of dairy cattle. Contagious pathogens spread from cow to cow, and environmental pathogens are present in the herd's environment, such as bedding materials, manure, and soil. Contagious pathogens *Staphylococcus aureus*, *Streptococcus agalactiae*, and S*treptococcus dysgalactiae* can easily adapt to the environment of the udder and spread from cow to cow during milking.[34]

Generally speaking, somatic cells are cells that make up the body. However, when it comes to the number of these cells in milk, it is difficult not to think that some form of deception is employed when government and the dairy industry use the number to refer to milk quality. With respect to the quality of milk, somatic cells are actually white blood cells (leukocytes, neutrophils, and macrophages), or more commonly, pus cells.

As usual, when it comes to food quality, the quality of milk, as indicated by the somatic cell count, is of concern to the government and the dairy industry, not because of issues with human health and the potential for disease

> Generally speaking, somatic cells are cells that make up the body.

exposure, but only because of the amount of money that the dairy industry stands to gain or lose. Milk with a low SCC means better milk products and a longer shelf life for the milk, both of which lead to greater profits or less loss. The health of the milk consumer is not an issue!

As the somatic cell count increases, so does the likelihood of the presence of disease, particularly mastitis. Mastitis is the inflammation of the udder. When the udder is inflamed, blood, mucus, and bacteria will be found in the milk of that particular cow; hence, the somatic cell count will increase considerably.

---

34 N. Sharma, N.K. Singh, M.S. Bhadwal, "Relationship of Somatic Cell Count and Mastitis: An Overview," *Asian-Australasian Journal of Animal Sciences* 24 (2011):429–438, https://1ref.us/1xp (accessed June 1, 2022); M.E. Alnakip, et al., "The Immunology of Mammary Gland of Dairy Ruminants between Healthy and Inflammatory Conditions," *Journal of Veterinary Medicine* (2014): 1–31, https://1ref.us/1xq (accessed June 1, 2022).

White blood cells called macrophages reside in the mammary gland. Their job is to identify the invading harmful bacteria. Once they find harmful bacteria, they then signal to other white blood cells and immune cells the presence of these bacteria.[35] Consequently, more immune cells are marshaled to the area of infection, and therefore, the SCC in milk increases. Phagocytic cells, namely, neutrophils and macrophages, after discovering the bacteria, will lock on and envelope the bacteria. The cells then proceed to destroy the bacteria by releasing enzymes that digest the bacteria. This process is known as phagocytosis.

In the European Union, China, New Zealand, Australia, Switzerland, and Canada, the legal bulk milk SCC (BMSCC) limit is 3–400,000 cells/mL; in South Africa and Brazil, 500,000 cells/mL; and in the USA, 750,000 cells/mL.[36] In the UK, an individual cow SCC of 100,000 or less indicates an "uninfected" cow, where there are no significant production losses due to subclinical mastitis. A threshold SCC of 200,000 would determine whether a cow is infected with mastitis. Cows infected with significant pathogens have an SCC of 300,000 or greater.[37] Cows with a result of greater than 200,000 are highly likely to be infected on at least one quarter in a year. It has been estimated that herds with a somatic cell count of 200,000,000 may have up to 15 percent of their cows infected. Somatic cell counts of 300,000,000 may have 25 percent of its cows infected. In the United Kingdom, if milk has an SCC of 400,000 or more, it is deemed unfit for human consumption.[38]

Somatic (pus) cell counts by state

The following are "average" somatic cell counts per milliliter of milk for each state in the U.S. in 2019.[39] The maximum number allowed is 750,000 per milliliter (1,000,000 per milliliter for goat's milk), which is well above the average. However, one must bear in mind that the average number of

---

35 "Somatic Cell Count and Mastitis," 429–438; "Dairy Ruminants," 1–31.

36 M. Alhussien and A. Dang, "Milk Somatic Cells, Factors Influencing Their Release, Future Prospects, and Practical Utility in Dairy Animals: An Overview," *Vet World* 11, no. 5 (2018): 562–577, https://1ref.us/1xo (accessed June 1, 2022).

37 "Mastitis In Cows: Somatic Cell Counts (SCCs)," AHDB, https://1ref.us/1xr (accessed June 1, 2022).

38 "Mastitis In Cows."

39 "Milk Somatic Cell Count from Dairy Herd Improvement Herds During 2021," CDCB, https://1ref.us/1xs (accessed June 1, 2022).

somatic cells includes days when the actual somatic count is well above 750,000! Of greater interest though, is the fact that the dairy industry's standard for milk that is fit for consumption is only 200,000 per milliliter! That being the case, only milk from a handful of states would qualify.

Alabama 303,000

Arizona 170,000

Arkansas 4351,000

California 191,000

Colorado 180,000

Connecticut 199,000

Delaware 242,000

Florida 223,000

Georgia 212,000

Idaho 148,000

Illinois 204,000

Indiana 191,000

Iowa 186,000

Kansas 208,000

Kentucky 257,000

Louisiana 301,000

Maine 179,000

Maryland 205,000

Massachusetts 199,000

Michigan 150,000

Minnesota 202,000

Mississippi 276,000

Missouri 258,000

Montana 183,000

Nebraska 193,000

Nevada 191,000

New Hampshire 154,000

New Jersey 262,000

New Mexico 175,000

New York 174,000

North Carolina 192,000

North Dakota 170,000

Ohio 180,000

Oklahoma 307,000

Oregon 153,000

Pennsylvania 189,000

Rhode island 190,000

South Carolina 251,000

South Dakota 202,000

Tennessee 274,000

Texas 194,000

Utah 157,000

Vermont 149,000

Virginia 204,000

Washington 158,000

West Virginia 206,000

Wisconsin 159,000

United States 187,000

In 2001, the SCC national average was 322,000,000.[40] Fortunately, the average SCC has dropped since 2001 to an average now of 179,000. The

---

40 "Somatic Cell Count 2021," CDCB.

drop may be due to any number of reasons ranging from vaccines to supplements to increased hygiene. If you want to make sense of and have a better understanding of these numbers, consider the average number of somatic cells in one cup of milk, enough to have with a bowl of cereal.

In Arkansas, the state with the highest SCC, 351,000, there would be an average of 83,042,000 somatic cells in the cup, whereas, in Idaho, the state with the lowest SCC, 148,000, there would be an average of 35,015,024 somatic cells floating around in your cup of milk.

Bacterial Counts

If the foregoing were not enough to turn your stomach, consider that in addition to the number of pus cells, milk also contains numerous bacteria floating around in it. Several tests are performed to determine the presence and number of bacteria per milliliter.

The Standard Plate Count (SPC) of a producer's raw milk samples gives an indication of the total number of aerobic (require oxygen) bacteria present in the milk at the time of pickup. Regulations require that bacteria counts of Grade "A" raw milk not exceed 100,000 SPC. In an ideal setting, the SPC could be 1000.[41]

In addition to somatic cells, aerobic bacteria, another type of bacteria, is also tested for coliform. Coliform bacteria are bacteria that are associated with fecal matter. Yes, milk is often contaminated with fecal matter due to the cow being soiled. The suggested limit is less than 50 per ml, though there is no regulatory limit, except in California, where the limit is to be less than 750 per ml.[42]

In addition to the contaminants above, milk will also contain antibiotic residue, viruses, etc. However, the greater problem is the health status of the cows that are producing milk. The health status is important because unhealthy cows will produce less milk, and their milk will have more bacteria, viruses, etc. Below are just a few of the diseases that afflict dairy cattle.

---

41 "Raw Milk Bacteria Tests—Sources and Causes of High Bacteria Counts," Cornell University, Dairy Foods Science Notes, https://1ref.us/1xt (accessed June 1, 2022).
42 "Raw Milk Bacteria Tests,"

Common Diseases of Cattle

Bovine Spongiform Encephalopathy (BSE) (also known as Mad Cow Disease)

BSE is a member of a group of fatal degenerative diseases known as Transmissible Spongiform Encephalopathies (TSE). These diseases affect the central nervous system. They attack the brain leaving characteristic holes, hence the name spongiform. Unlike a large number of diseases, BSE is, and TSEs in general, quite puzzling in the way they are transmitted. It is resistant to extreme temperatures, ultraviolet, and ionizing radiation. It is even resistant to formaldehyde and glutaraldehyde.

BSE exists in two forms: Classical (C-type) and atypical (L-type or H-type). The incubation period for classical BSE is three to six years. This form of BSE is believed to be acquired from cattle ingesting the BSE causative agent in contaminated feed. Such contaminated feed would be derived from meat and bone meal of rendered BSE-infected cattle.[43]

Atypical forms of BSE can occur spontaneously in all cattle of any age. It appears that cattle older than eight years of age are more prone to the disease than younger cattle. Interestingly, the atypical type does not appear to be brought on by the ingestion of contaminated feed as is the case with classical BSE but appears spontaneously.[44]

BSE-infected cattle initially lose coordination, stumble, and eventually are unable to walk or stand. They lose weight as well as have a decrease in the production of milk. Behaviorally, the animals display nervousness and aggression. The incubation period is two to eight years. Once symptoms develop. Death usually occurs in a few months.

The disease was spread to cattle in Britain in feed consisting of brains, meat, bone meal, and by-products of sheep that were infected with a scrapie-like organism. Scrapie is a neurological disease that affects sheep; it is a member of the TSEs. This disease is common in sheep in the U.S. The use of meat, bone meal, and animal by-products for feed from cud-chewing animals, such as sheep, is a widespread practice in the U.S. and abroad. Cows normally eat grass and vegetation. Unfortunately, it is a widespread practice in this age of modern meat to feed cows the ground-up flesh of other animals as a means of generating revenue from the

---

43 "Bovine Spongiform Encephalopathy (BSE)," USDA Animal and Plant Health Inspection Service, June 2, 2020, https://1ref.us/1xu (accessed June 1, 2022).
44 "BSE."

billions of pounds of waste from inedible portions of animal carcasses. This product consists of a variety of animals that have had a number of health problems. You cannot expect to have healthy animals when they are fed the flesh of sick ones! In the United States, efforts to minimize the spread of BSE were put into place by banning the use of brains and spinal columns from the rendering process. Per the USDA mammalian protein may be prohibited the inclusion of mammalian protein in feed for cattle and other ruminants since 1997, that does not include mammalian fat, carbohydrates, collagen, calcium, and other minerals. The prohibition of high-risk tissue materials in all animal feed since 2009 is almost comical because prions have been found in other places in the body.

The health issue that humans face is to what extent, if any, that BSE is spread to humans. We know for a certainty that BSE is found in the brain and spinal cord. However, BSE is also found in meat and meat products.[45] A greater concern, however, for this book is whether or not BSE is found in milk and milk products. For years, there was a denial that BSE is found in milk. A study from 2008 showed that prions, the causative agent of BSE and a similar disease in sheep, were found in the milk of sheep.[46] If prions are in the milk of sheep, it makes sense that prions are in the milk of cows affected with Mad Cow Disease. It was also in 2008 that scientists working for the Swiss firm Alicon discovered prions in the milk of cows.[47]

When the mad Cow outbreak happened in Britain, not only did they kill the cows, but they also destroyed the milk from suspected cows. Given that prions can exist in 1,000-degree temperatures and require being exposed to temperatures in excess of 900 degrees for several hours to be effectively killed, the prion will not in the least be affected by the pasteurization process of milk.[48]

There has been an ever-growing concern about the possible relationship between BSE and its equivalent in humans, ™Creutzfeldt-Jacob Disease (CJD). CJD had been a disease that affected older people; however, in Britain, an alarming number of people in their twenties and younger

---

45 "Fast Facts—Bovine Spongiform Encephalopathy (BSE)," The Center for Food Security and Public Health, Iowa State University, https://1ref.us/1xv (accessed June 1, 2022).
46 T. Konold, et al., "Evidence of Scrapie Transmission via Milk," *BMC Veterinary Research* 4 (2008): 14, https://1ref.us/1xw (accessed June 1, 2022).
47 C. Mercer, "Study Highlights Milk BSE Risk," Dairyreporter.com, https://1ref.us/1xx (accessed June 1, 2022).
48 "What Are Prions?" Virginia DWR, https://1ref.us/1xy (accessed June 1, 2022).

have died recently with CJD. As early as 1997, it was reported that a vegetarian had been diagnosed with the new "variant" Creutzfeldt-Jacob disease (CJD).[49] Scientists feared that this person contracted CJD from contaminated milk and cheese. There have been several other cases of people in their twenties diagnosed with this same form of CJD. There may very well be many more cases of it in the world that have gone undetected because of the symptoms that appear to rival those of Parkinson's and Alzheimer's.

One would think that the government would have the health of its citizens as its top priority; however, such is not the case with the USDA. The USDA exists for the viability and benefit of the meat and dairy industry. It is concerned about their profits, not the health of U.S. citizens. It could care less about the health of consumers. With respect to the health of the U.S. citizens, the only health that the USDA is interested in is the health of your bank account to purchase food items from the meat and dairy industry. Think I am wrong??? Consider this—Would it not be beneficial to test every cow for BSE? Would not every citizen want to know that the meat and milk they consume and give to their children is from cows that have been tested and found free of BSE? Creekstone Farms in Kansas started a firestorm when it went public, stating that it wanted to test every cow for BSE that it slaughters. Creekstone is a small slaughterhouse by modern-day standards; they slaughter approximately 300,000 cattle per year.

> *Creekstone Farms seem to be proud of the products that carry their name and wanted to assure the public that their products were from cows that were tested for BSE.*

I applaud the efforts of Creekstone Farms. They seem to be proud of the products that carry their name and wanted to assure the public that their products were from cows that were tested for BSE. The USDA is the only distributor of the kits. After investing half a million dollars to start the testing, the USDA refused to give Creekstone the kits to test for BSE. Why did they refuse? The USDA maintains that the testing is not necessary and would give Creekstone an unfair advantage in marketing its meat as free of Mad Cow! What was really happening was that the egos in the USDA were in the way of the best interests of the consumer. The

---

49 Charles Arthur, "Vegetarian, 24, Gets CJD," Independent, https://1ref.us/1xz (accessed June 1, 2022).

USDA had entrenched itself in a position that many consumer groups, and even members of Congress saw as horrible policy.

Fortunately, Creekstone did not give up their legal fight and allow themselves to be bullied by the USDA and their parade of lawyers. After a multi-year legal fight, Creekstone won its battle with the USDA and was allowed to use rapid test kits to screen their cattle for BSE.[50]

The USDA lost due to its hypocrisy and double standard. On the one hand, USDA can't argue that the test kits are useful for diagnosing and managing BSE when used by USDA, but the same exact tests are "worthless" when used by a private company. The test gives the consumer a hint of a margin of safety in that the cattle were tested for BSE; however, the test is not a guarantee that the tested cattle are free of BSE. The amount it costs per animal is around $20.

One would think, one would hope, that the USDA would have the same concern for the health of the consumer as Creekstone. Why does not the USDA test for BSE in EVERY cow that is slaughtered like Creekstone??? Profits, profits, profits!!! Given that the cost of the test is $20, and results can be had in a few hours, it would cost the industry about $600,000,000 to test the 30+ million cattle that are slaughtered each year. Needless to say, the meat industry does not want to "waste" more than half a billion dollars testing for BSE, especially if it increases the likelihood of discovering many more cases of BSE than has been discovered by the current scientifically statistical method that it currently employs in testing only 25,000 cattle per year, less than 1/10 of 1 percent of the cattle that are slaughtered every year.[51] Given these numbers, it is easy for the USDA to say that it has found no evidence of BSE, especially, if the program suspects that an animal has BSE, but does not inspect it, but instead orders that it be sent to be rendered (processed for animal food). It is also suspicious that the number of cattle tested dropped from 40,000 to 25,000. Could it be that the USDA is catering to pressure from the meat industry???

Bovine Leukemia Virus (BLV)
Bovine Leukemia Virus was discovered in the late 1960s. It is an oncogenic (cancer-causing) retrovirus. A retrovirus is a virus that uses the enzyme

---

50 "Court Ruled Creekstone Farms Allowed to Use Rapid Test Kits to Screen Their Cattle for BSE," Press Release, May 29, 2007, https://1ref.us/1y0 (accessed June 1, 2022).
51 "BSE Surveillance Information Center," USDA, https://1ref.us/1y1 (accessed June 1, 2022).

known as reverse transcriptase to translate its genetic information into DNA. That DNA can then integrate into the host cell's DNA. When integration is complete, the virus can hijack the host cell's components to make additional viral particles. BLV attacks a special type of white blood cells known as lymphocytes. As these cells increase in number, they can lead to leukemia and a condition in which tumors form and invade organs in the body.

BLV is becoming of great concern. It is distributed worldwide. Unfortunately, the U.S. has the dubious distinction of having the second-highest concentration of BLV in the world! More than 80 percent of the dairy herds in the United States are infected with BLV.[52] **In addition, BLV is so prevalent that nearly half (46.5%) of all dairy cows have BLV and this number is likely to continue to increase.**[53]

The USDA does not test for BLV prior to slaughter. As you may have guessed, many of the cattle infected with BLV are sent to slaughter and have become hamburgers! The main concern for the USDA is the money lost due to decreased milk production from cows with BLV.

The bovine leukemia virus has been classified in the same group as the Human T-cell Leukemia/Lymphotropic virus type 1 (HTLV-1), which is known to cause leukemia and lymphomas in humans.[54] A study was done on infant chimpanzees that were fed raw milk from cows infected with BLV. These chimps developed leukemia and Pneumocyctis carinii pneumonia. What was astounding about this is that Pneumocyctis carinii pneumonia had never been reported in chimpanzees, and it is the very same type of pneumonia that some people with AIDS die from! Given this, the "experts" will still tell us that there is nothing to fear!!!

When BLV was isolated in 1969, the tests and technology available at that time were not able to detect BLV in humans. In order to pacify any fears the public could legitimately have and to keep the beef and dairy industry alive, the USDA concluded that BLV was not transmissible

---

52 V. Ruggiero, et al., "Controlling Bovine Leukemia Virus In Dairy Herds by Identifying and Removing Cows with Highest Proviral Load and Lymphocyte Counts," *Journal of Science* 102:9165–9175, https://1ref.us/1y2 (accessed June 1, 2022).
53 R. LaDronka, et al., "Prevalence of Bovine Leukemia Virus Antibodies In US Dairy Cattle," *Veterinary Medicine International,* https://1ref.us/1y3 (accessed June 1, 2022).
54 N. Sagata, Y. Ikawa, "BLV and HTLV-I: Their Unique Genomic Structures and Evolutionary Relationship," Princess Takamatsu Symposium 15 (1984):229–40, https://1ref.us/1y4 (accessed June 1, 2022).

to humans. The technology employed in those days was such that they missed 70 percent of the bovine cases, so it is not surprising that human cases were not found. However, that is where common sense comes in. If the virus is found in a cow and its milk, then when a human consumes the cow or its milk, it makes sense the virus will be found in the human. Such a conclusion does not require rocket science. However, it does require a willingness to investigate, rather than a willingness to protect an industry.

It took thirty-five years, but interest in the presence of BLV in humans, the study was resurrected. A study was conducted to investigate whether or not humans could have BLV. Unlike the testing a few decades earlier, which relied on agar gel immunodiffusion and complement fixation assays which failed to find BLV, this time researchers used a far more sensitive technique for finding BLV, immunoblotting was used to test the sera for antibodies to the BLV capsid antigen. In 2004, in the journal *AIDS Research and Human Retroviruses* in which researchers, chief of whom was Dr. Gertrude Buehring at the University of California at Berkeley, discovered that a significant proportion of Americans may have antibodies to BLV due to consuming beef and or dairy products. BLV infected cells are in the blood of cattle and the milk of cows.

Dr. Buehring and her colleagues took blood samples from 257 people, most of whom were women, and tested them for the presence of BLV antibodies. They found that at least one antibody of the four isotypes to the BLV capsid was in 74 percent of the human sera tested.[55] If those numbers hold true for the general population, it is chilling to think of the millions of people who have the infection and are likely candidates for cancer.

There is undoubtedly a connection between BLV and its expression on humans. The parts of the country with the highest rates of BLV-infected cattle have higher rates of human leukemia. In Iowa, the counties with the highest BLV infections also had the highest rates of acute lymphoblastic leukemia. Studies have also shown that milk consumption is associated with the development of malignant lymphomas.

---

55 G. Buehring, S. Philpott, and K. Choi, "Human Have Antibodies Reactive with Bovine Leukemia Virus," *AIDS Research and Human Retroviruses* 19, no. 12 (2003): 1105–1113, https://1ref.us/1y5 (accessed June 2, 2022).

Bovine Immunodeficiency Virus (BIV, also known as Cow AIDS!!!)
BIV, like HIV, is probably one of the most politically influenced diseases on record. BIV is found in dairy and beef cattle in the United States, Canada, Costa Rica, and Europe. It is literally found in cattle all over the world! However, it seems that the only people who know about it are the scientists who perform experiments with it. Politics and corporate money have been successful in keeping information about this disease out of the media.

The discovery of BIV is not recent; in fact, it was discovered in 1972![56] Unfortunately, at the time it was discovered, attention was focused on BLV. Interest was not directed toward BIV until HIV came along. BIV is a bovine lentivirus (any of a group of retroviruses [RNA viruses]) that is genetically, structurally, and antigenically related to HIV type1![57] BIV is found in the blood and milk of cattle, it is also found in the semen of bulls. This virus may impair the immune system of cattle, just as the AIDS virus impairs the immune system of humans. It was soon discovered that cattle infected with BIV were also found to be infected with BLV as well. BIV and BLV can cross species lines and infect other types of animals such as sheep, goats, and even chimpanzees. BIV has even been found in humans! One major concern is that this disease, especially mild cases of it, would be difficult to detect in dairy cattle because of BIV testing sensitivity and specificity, in addition to the increased likelihood of these cattle being removed from the herd and sent to slaughter due to the reduction in the production of milk and a high amount of blood in their milk.

The "experts" will tell you that this disease poses no threat to humans!!! That may be what they say now, but what will they be saying in the next year or two??? They want you to take comfort in the thought that pasteurization kills many types of microorganisms. However, pasteurization is not without its flaws, even when done correctly! It is possible that pasteurization may actually break the virus into fragments that could pose an even greater danger.

---

56 "Bovine Immunodeficiency Virus," *Methods In Enzymology* (2019), https://1ref.us/1y6 (accessed June 2, 2022).
57 O. Straub and D. Levy, "Bovine Immunodeficiency Virus and Analogies with Human Immunodeficiency Virus," *Leukemia* 13 (1999): s106–s109, https://1ref.us/1y8 (accessed June 2, 2022).

Pyemia (pus in the blood)
Animals with pyemia have cocci, bacillus coli, or other pus-producing organisms in their blood. In addition to the various hemorrhages formed as in septicemia, abscesses form in various organs of the body.

Septicemia (poison blood)
Septicemia is characterized by destructive changes in the blood. The blood becomes deep brown in color, noncoagulable, and is full of bacteria. The spleen becomes larger and contains black blood. Animals with septicemia have hemorrhages in the heart, lungs, liver, and kidneys. They are not inclined to move and are not aware of their surroundings.

Hemorrhagic Septicemia
Hemorrhagic Septicemia is also called cattle disease, barbone, and pasteurellosis bovina. This disease is highly fatal and is caused by the microorganism <u>Bacterium bovisepticum</u>, which belongs to the same group of cocci-bacilli as those which cause chicken cholera, swine plague, and rabbit septicemia. Hemorrhagic septicemia manifests itself in various forms, as described below.

Superficial or cutaneous
Animals suffering from this form of the disease have difficulty in breathing, eating, swallowing, and have swollen throats and tongues. They also have a loss of appetite and secrete less milk.

Pulmonary
Animals suffering from this form exhibit the same symptoms as those suffering from croupous pneumonia. They have difficulty breathing, severe diarrhea, followed by weakness. The animal dies within 24–36 hours.

Pectoral
There is a free flow of saliva from the mouth. This form is 80-90 percent fatal.

Lesions of Hemorrhagic Septicemia
Hemorrhagic areas in the subcutaneous, subserous, and muscular tissues, lymph glands, and the viscera vary in size anywhere from a small dot to the size of a nickel or more. The superficial form appears as a doughy tumefaction of the skin in the area of the throat, neck, and even legs. Mucous membranes and submucous tissues of the mouth, tongue, and throat are greatly inflamed, thickened, and filled with serum. The lymph

glands swell and are also filled with serum. Throughout the muscular system, there are hemorrhagic areas.

Bovine Tuberculosis

Tuberculosis is caused by *Tubercle bacillus*, specifically, *Mycobacterium bovis*, which is transmissible to humans and other animals. Once it is inside of the body, T. bacillus organisms will start to embed in the tissues where they will grow, multiply, and excrete substances that will act as poisons and will lead to the formation of a tubercle or nodule. The stomach, intestines, ovaries, uterus, diaphragm, spleen, liver, walls of the abdomen, testicles, brain, spinal cord, and the mesenteric glands are affected. It is rarely found in the bones. The tubercles or nodules range in size from a speck to the size of an egg.

T. bacillus may enter the body by inhalation into the lungs or drinking the milk of a cow with tuberculosis, and the mother may pass it on to her fetus. The milk becomes thin and watery and is mixed with flakes and tubercle bacilli. Animals may abort, experience convulsions, unconsciousness, and paralysis. Death usually results from exhaustion after an illness lasting a few months to even a few years.

Variola (cowpox)

Affects the udders and teats, generally with pustular eruptions. The animals secrete less milk and have an elevated temperature.

Actinomycosos

Actinomycosos is also known as lumpy jaw, big jaw, and wooden tongue. It is caused by actinomyces fungus. The disease is commonly found on the bones of the jaw, parotid gland, and in the area of the throat. The disease may attack the tongue and manifest itself in the form of a tumor in the mouth and throat. In the generalized condition, the muscular tissue, liver, brain, and spleen are affected. The disease may start in the bone marrow or in the covering of the bone. The animal may have difficulty breathing and may die from suffocation due to the presence of a tumor in the pharynx.

Anthrax

Anthrax is caused by a bacterium, which has spores that are highly resistant to heat and can remain viable for extended periods of time. The disease may begin in the skin, lungs, or in the intestines. Death usually occurs as a result of the bacteria multiplying and producing toxins.

Anthrax peracutus (apoplectiform)
The animal dies suddenly as if it experienced a severe stroke.

Anthrax acutis without external swellings
Animals with this form of the disease have increased temperature, muscle tumors, chills, and weakness. If the disease reaches the intestine, the animal will experience severe pain; the stools, which are normally firm, will become soft and covered with blood and mucous. The nose, mouth, rectum, and vagina may discharge blood due to ruptured vessels. Death occurs in one or two days.

Lesions
Lesions occur in the fatty layer under the skin but are often overlooked because of the skin's healthy appearance. The spleen is often two to five times its normal size.

Pseudoencephalomalacia
This is a highly fatal disease of cattle marked by edema of the brain, blindness, and the inability to stand.

Malignant Catarrh
The disease starts with a chill that later develops into a fever. The skin becomes hot and dry, and various muscles begin to quiver. Constipation is evident initially but later changes to diarrhea. A diphtheric membrane is formed on the mucous membranes of the mouth, nose, and throat. The animal may experience difficulty in breathing and perhaps even suffocation because of the croupous membranes which form in the throat. The horns of the animal can be damaged and destroyed because of inflammation of the horn core. Lesions of the eye result in inflammation of the iris and permanent cloudiness of the cornea. The kidneys and the bladder become inflamed, which leads to difficulty in urination. The disease finally leads to dementia, delirium, spasms, convulsions, and paralysis. The disease is 50-90 percent fatal.

Malignant Edema
This disease is also known as Gangrenous septicemia. It is basically an acute inflammatory disease.

Foot and Mouth Disease
Foot and mouth disease may attack the same animals repeatedly and is highly contagious. The feet of the animal become sensitive and sore,

causing the animal to lie down continually in an attempt to rest its feet. This action then causes the animal to develop decubitis ulcers on its body as a result of being in one position too long. This disease may manifest itself internally prior to being seen externally. The animal may die from choking due to paralysis of the throat, suffocation due to paralysis of the lungs, or even from a heart attack due to paralysis of the heart muscle. The milk from animals suffering from this disease causes fatal diarrhea in suckling calves and pigs.

Borna Disease
This is a fatal enzootic encephalitis of cattle caused by a virus.

Sporadic Bovine Encephalomyelitis
This is a viral encephalomyelitis with pleuritis, which affects cattle in the U.S. Affected animals suffer from dullness, hard breathing, diarrhea, and a staggering gait.

Southern Cattle Fever (Texas fever)
Acute
The red blood cells are destroyed at an extraordinary rate. Up to ten pounds of blood can be destroyed in a twenty-four-hour period. The debris that results from this destruction has to be converted into bile or excreted from the animal's system. Often the result is death due to the excess load placed upon the liver.

Mild
The spleen, liver, and gall bladder become grossly enlarged. Prior to death, the feces that the affected animal excretes is soft and filled with bile.

Blackleg
The general symptoms of this disease are similar to those resembling acute infection or those of bacterial diseases.

Necrotic Stomatitis (calf diphtheria)
This disease is caused by *Bacillus necrophorus* and is a causative factor in foot rot, diphtheric inflammation of the small intestine of calves, necrosis of the heart in cattle, multiple liver abscesses, embolic necrosis of the lung, disseminated liver necrosis, diphtheria of the uterus and vagina. The general symptoms are lack of energy, weakness, excessive salivation, elevated temperature, and a swollen tongue.

Chronic Bacterial Dysentery
Initially, the animal may experience moderate diarrhea, which eventually becomes excessive, leading to serious weight loss. The animal becomes anemic, emaciated, and develops weakness in its muscles. Death is generally the result of emaciation and chronic diarrhea.

Pearl Disease
Tuberculosis of the mesentery and peritoneum.

Bovine Encephalitis
Encephalitis that is caused by the psittacosis-lymphogranuloma venerum group.

Infectious bovine rhinotracheitis (IBR)
Infectious bovine rhinotracheitis (IBR) is a viral disease caused by bovine herpesvirus 1 (BHV-1) that can also cause a mild venereal infection in cattle or a brain infection in calves. IBR is a highly contagious disease of the upper respiratory tract and can lead to pneumonia. The clinical signs of the disease are nasal discharge, fever, and conjunctivitis. Acute disease in dairy cattle is usually accompanied by a severe and prolonged drop in milk productionthe main concern of dairymen and women!

Cattle Farcy
This disease is caused by infection with *Nocardia Farcinica*. The subcutaneous tissue and organs of the affected animal are filled with cheesy nodules.

Carbuncular Fever
This is a form of anthrax in which swellings of the skin become gangrenous.

Shipping Fever
This disease is caused by *Pasteurella haemolytica* in conjunction with a virus when the animal's resistance is lowered as a result of stress.

Bovine Leptospirosis
Caused primarily by *Leptospira interrogans*, serogroup *pomona*, affected animals will suffer jaundice, fever, and anemia.

Polioencephalomalacia
Polioencephalomalacia is a common neurological disease. It is an acute disease characterized by dullness, head pressing, blindness, opisthotonos,

nystagmus, and paddling movements of the limbs. Convulsions and death soon follow.

Malignant Lymphoma of Cattle
This disease is marked by fatal abnormal and progressive growth of some, in some cases, all of the lymph nodes.

Bovine Ulcerative Mammillitis
This herpes viral disease of milking cows manifests itself with ulcerative lesions on the teats and occasionally on the udders.

Necrobacillosis
Infection with Fusobacterium necrophorum is the cause of this disease. It causes diphtheria with abscesses and areas of necrosis.

Paravaccinia (Milker's Nodules)
This is a cutaneous disease of cattle and can be spread to humans by simple contact.

Parasites of the Gastrointestinal Tract of Cattle
Gongylonema pulchurum
This worm is a common parasite in the esophagus.

Twisted stomach worm (Haemonchus Contortus)
This worm causes anemia, weakness, excessive thirst, and diarrhea. It is usually found in the fourth stomach of cattle.

Encysted stomach worm (Ostertagia)
This worm causes anemia, weakness, excessive thirst, and diarrhea. It is also found in cysts on the wall of the fourth stomach of cattle.

Paramphistomum cervi
This fluke is usually found in the rumen and reticulum.

Tapeworms

Tapeworms can grow more than forty feet in length. They cause emaciation in calves. The beef tapeworm is the most common one found in humans. They cause illness by encroaching on the host's food supply, producing waste material, and by obstructing the intestinal tract.

Tapeworms can grow more than forty feet in length.

Taenia saginata (Beef tapeworm)
These range in length from thirteen to thirty feet. The larval stage is found in the flesh of cattle. The adult worms can be found in humans.

Cystircercus bovis
This is the larval form of Taenia saginata.

Roundworms

Hookworms
These cause symptoms similar to those of infection with stomach worms. The bites of hookworms can cause inflammation, which in turn renders the intestine more susceptible to infection.

Slender roundworms (Trichostrongylus)
These worms cause severe gastroenteritis.

Ascaris ovis
These are immature specimens of Ascaris lumbricoides.

Chabertia ovina
Known as the large-mouth bowel worm, it is parasitic in the colon.

Parasites of the Liver and Lung of cattle

Tapeworm cysts (Multiceps multiceps, Coernurus cerebralis)
Cattle ingest the eggs. The embryos then migrate to the liver, brain, and lungs, where they form cysts of various sizes.

Echinococcus granulosus (hydatid worm)
These are only one-quarter of an inch long. The larval form is found in cattle, sheep, and pigs. The size of the cysts formed depends upon what organ is invaded. Cysts the size of a football have been found in humans as a result of infections of up to twenty years in duration. This can be fatal in humans.

Lung worms (Dictyocaulus viviparus)
These are up to four inches long and are found in the bronchial tubes.

Parasites of the Blood of Cattle
Flukes (Schistosoma bovis)
Causes the disease Schistosomiasis. They live in the blood vessels and cause blood to be in the urine.

Piroplasma bigeminum
These live in the blood and attack the red blood cells and cause Texas Fever.

Pathogens Present in Animals and Animal Products Which Can Cause Disease in Humans

Clostridium botulin
This microorganism produces several types of toxins which affect the nervous system and are among perhaps the deadliest poisons known to man. Symptoms occur twenty-four to forty-eight hours after ingestion. Death occurs as a result of paralysis of the muscles which control breathing. Approximately two out of every three cases are fatal.

Clostridium perfringes
This microorganism causes abdominal pain and diarrhea, which occurs eight to twenty-two hours after it is ingested.

Leptospira interrogans
These can cause a wide range of problems and can be fatal. Jaundice is a common feature of the severe forms of the disease.

Listeria monocytogenes
This microorganism is common in the milk and blood of animals. It produces septicemia and encephalomyelitis in lower animals. In humans, it produces meningoencephalitis, meningitis, perinatal septicemia, and other disorders.

Salmonella
This is one of the most common culprits involved in food poisoning. Symptoms of gastrointestinal upset occur twelve to twenty-four hours after ingestion. There are over 2,000 types of salmonella!!!

Bacillus megatherium
Causes souring in beef.

Staphyloccus Aureus
Symptoms occur two to six hours after ingestion. In humans, these microorganisms have been associated with impetigo, carbuncles, septicemia, pneumonia, and endocarditis.

It is important to note that cattle suffer from a number of cancers throughout the body as well. Perhaps the most common cancer they have is eye cancer. However, cattle also have cancers ranging from skin cancer to cancer of the lymph nodes.

Chapter 3

SLAUGHTERHOUSE

The Dead-End Road for Happy Cows

Happy Cows?
Once upon a time, in a land flowing with milk and opportunity, the major animals currently being used for food—cows, chickens, hogs, and turkeys—were allowed to roam freely on the family farm and feed on the tall, green grass. Here they would get plenty of exercise and fresh air. Furthermore, they would eat foods that were a natural part of their diet. However, today, things are vastly different. Animals are now raised on corporate farms and feedlots. Animals have become "products," "units" to be fed into the industrial and the corporate computers to determine the profit margin for the current period.

Animals are no longer viewed as animals, beings with senses, emotions, feelings, etc. Instead, they are now viewed as inanimate objects, the products of manufacturing. It is a direct result of this mentality that man has sought to take control of animals even prior to conception, to the point where their bodies have been mechanically ravaged, and their flesh is slowly being digested in the stomach of some unsuspecting person.

In order to make animals "products," Satan has, via humans, sought to control and manipulate virtually every aspect of an animals' existence prior to conception and up to the point of death. Females are exposed to a wide range of powerful hormones such as chlorandinone acetate, melengestrol acetate, and medroxyprogesterone acetate, which are used to control estrus and ovulation in sheep and cattle. By manipulating estrus and ovulation, artificial insemination and earlier rebreeding become viable tools in increasing the "bottom line" of the meat industry. However, these procedures are not without costs as they often result in inducing shock and premature death.

On some farms where artificial insemination is practiced, males are used to detect females that are ready to breed. Unfortunately for these males, they are not allowed to copulate with the females they find ready to breed. In order to frustrate them in their attempt to copulate with the willing females, various bizarre devices have been employed to keep the male's penis from entering the female. One such device does not allow the penis to extend naturally and forces it to remain within its sheath. This results in pain as well as infection. Another device that is employed calls for the removal of the penis. Yet still another device routes the penis to exit to the side at the flank. Do these methods sound natural?

Since every square inch of space is utilized on corporate farms with large numbers of animals, unnatural adjustments and other manipulations must be made in order to keep production costs down. For instance, slaughterhouses are now known as packing plants. Daily, people with "sophisticated" palates are seated in expensive gourmet restaurants chicly ordering veal parmigiana. It sounds so sophisticated and elitist. Our taste buds have been altered to such an extent that we take delight in and crave the flesh of a sickly baby calf as our minds ignore the horror this creature endured during its truly short life. However, the name does not negate the horrible treatment and abuse the animals that provide their flesh for this item have to endure.

Many veal cows come from dairy stock. In order to keep dairy cows producing milk, they must become pregnant repeatedly. When these dairy cows give birth to females, they are eventually added to the dairy herd. However, when a male is born, it is used for veal since a male cow cannot produce milk, and because it is from the dairy line, its flesh is not well suited for beef. Literally, within twenty-four hours after birth, the baby male calf is taken away from its mother and placed in a stall so small that it cannot move around in it. This will be its home until it either dies or is killed. By being taken so soon from its mother, many calves go into shock and die. Deprived of its mother's milk, the calves are given a milk substitute that is high in fat and lacks nutritional value. This substance is designed to make them gain as much weight as fast as possible. The calves are not given any grains, straw, or hay for fear of their flesh turning darker because of the content of iron in the grains.

The premature removal from the mother, the unnatural diet, and the lack of exercise combine to exact a heavy toll on calves used for veal. It is not unusual for 30 percent or more to die prior to being sent to slaughter. Many more would die if they were kept much longer. Some veal calves are sent to market as early as one month of age. The majority, however, are sent to market between three and four months of age. If they waited any longer to take them to market, many would die from their anemic and weakened state.

In an attempt to decrease muscle development and increase weight gain, calves that are destined to become veal are not allowed to exercise at all. Chained to small cages, they are not even able to turn around, stretch their legs, or even lie down in a natural position. To decrease their restlessness, they are kept in total darkness. Respiratory and intestinal diseases are common among these calves. They also suffer from chronic diarrhea as a result of being fed exclusively a liquid diet, no solid food whatsoever, of powdered skim milk, growth stimulants, antibiotics, vitamins, and mold inhibitors. This also serves to keep them from succumbing to their weakened state and to keep them alive long enough to get them to slaughter and to make a profit.

Modern meat animals are raised on farms that are tantamount to twentieth-century biological manufacturing entities. These animals are kept under crowded conditions. There are many problems which result because of these crowded conditions. Believe it or not, animals are social creatures, and as such, when they are placed under unnatural conditions such as crowding, they experience a great deal of stress. Animals are affected by stress in many ways. For instance, as the level of stress increases, the animals become more susceptible to disease due to the lowering of their resistance. Also, under crowded conditions, diseases can spread easily and rapidly to every animal in the group. Just one diseased animal can infect the entire group in a brief period of time.

Cattle are often branded with hot irons, have their horns cut off, and are even castrated without anything to numb the pain! However, the cruelest act that animals must endure is that of being killed! After being milked for

> *Believe it or not, animals are social creatures, and as such, when they are placed under unnatural conditions such as crowding, they experience a great deal of stress.*

upwards of five to six years, being artificially impregnated as many times as possible, and producing six to seven gallons of milk each day, death is a welcomed event.

From Happy Cow to Hamburger

When I was younger, about five or six years of age, my aunt took me to our neighborhood butcher shop, where she always purchased her chickens. This was the first time I had ever stepped foot in the place, and it was a day that I will never forget! I was barely able to see over the large wooden counter as my aunt picked out the chicken that she wanted. What I saw horrified me! The butcher went over to the cage that contained the chicken that my aunt wanted and grabbed it from the dirty cage. All of the other chickens in the cage started running all over the place, screaming and flapping their wings excitedly as though they were scared to death.

Little did I know that they knew what was going to happen to them. The chicken that the butcher grabbed seemed really frightened. It began flapping its wings wildly and pecking the butcher's hand in a futile attempt to escape its inevitable fate. Unfortunately for the chicken, it was not able to get away. The butcher then grabbed the chicken firmly with one hand and, with the other hand, picked up a large, sharp knife and proceeded to chop off the chicken's head!

I could not believe what I saw! Even after the chicken's head was completely cut off, it still kept moving wildly; even the body kept making wild movements. I was horrified at the sight! Words cannot describe the horror that filled my juvenile mind! It seemed too barbaric to be real. It was so cruel, so unreal. How could a person do that? I could not understand how the butcher could do what he did. I also understood why the other chickens in the cage were so frantic as well; they saw everything that I did!

Up to this point in my life, I had never associated meats with bloody, dead animals—I just thought of meats as being just another type of food. I had no idea that what I thought were cute little animals had to be killed in order to provide us with meat. It has been many years since I witnessed that awful event in my neighborhood butcher shop. Now that I am older, I still reflect on that day and still see that poor little chicken getting its head cut off. That event still fills me with emotion. Knowing that animals are still being unmercifully murdered just for the sake of providing meat nauseates me.

As I began doing the research for this book, one of the things that I had planned was to make a visit to a modern slaughterhouse. People have told me over the years how terrible slaughterhouses were. They would tell me what I thought were gross exaggerations about the smell of the slaughterhouses, the blood on the floor, the unsanitary conditions, etc. What they were telling me seemed a bit too hard to believe. In my naive mind, I thought that slaughterhouses were as clean as any hospital operating room, hence my difficulty in accepting the stories I was told. At any rate, I made it a point to find out for myself what a modern slaughterhouse was really like so that I may accurately share that information with you.

Fortunately, I was not alone in my desire to visit a slaughterhouse. My good friend and fellow health enthusiast from Oakland, Milton Mills, now Stanford medical school alum Dr. Milton Mills, who appears in the documentary *What the Health*, and I teamed up and decided to go to a slaughterhouse together to see for ourselves what really went on in them. The first slaughterhouse that we visited was not too terribly friendly toward having visitors, especially those who asked a lot of questions, and especially because two Black men were asking the questions! We were not allowed inside this slaughterhouse to witness the slaughtering of cattle. However, the manager of the slaughterhouse informed us that because of the small size of their operation, they slaughtered cattle by hand and did not have the automated equipment found in larger, more modern slaughterhouses.

The next slaughterhouse that Milton and I visited was a medium-sized automated plant. When we arrived, we asked if we could tour the facility. A quick call was made, and in short order, we were met by the owner. The owner, a young, "cool," relaxed white guy, was very friendly and hospitable. We introduced ourselves, and Milton told him rather candidly that we would like to see the goings-on in the slaughterhouse. The owner was not the least bit intimidated or hostile to our request. Milton and I must have looked like quintessential non-threatening young academics. Perhaps it was Milton's argyle sweater that made the difference! I think Milton and I were both taken aback at how relaxed he was, especially when compared to the reception we had at the first slaughterhouse. The guy was incredibly open and transparent. The interaction that he had with the workers was much like that of a co-worker than that of a boss. He did not try to hide or sugarcoat anything. The employees were a friendly group of guys who welcomed our presence with smiles. However, I could not fathom, let alone understand, how people could be smiling in such a sickly, gory place. No doubt there had to be an adjustment in their mental and emotional state in order to work in such a setting. The owner warned us about what we would see and gave us carte blanche to tour his slaughterhouse. We did not have to sign any forms, we were not given a time limit, and we were not even asked what we would do. I was amazed at the amount of freedom we were given to move about the place. The owner undoubtedly felt that he had nothing to hide and seemed to even take pride in his business.

Upon entering the grounds of this slaughterhouse, the smell of dust, urine, and manure filled the air! There was a large, fenced area, commonly called the "yard." This area was sectioned off in such a manner that it forced the entering herd of cattle into a more manageable and desirable single-file line, the line of death. The cows were packed in close one behind one another in this line of death. It was a sad sight for me, for I knew that in just a few short moments, these animals would be dead. Even though I knew that these animals were going to be killed, I was not at all prepared for the way in which their fate would be sealed.

In order to get to the actual slaughterhouse, we had to walk along a small bridge, which was just a few feet above the line of cattle. As I looked down on the cattle, I could not help but notice the fear and anxiety they were experiencing. They appeared scared, jittery, and nervous. They had a nervous energy similar to that of someone experiencing intense fear. It was a bizarre feeling to look into the eyes of an innocent animal that was just minutes away from a horrible death. I felt powerless. I wanted to buy all of the cows in the line and set them free, but I couldn't. There was nothing that I could do to stop their impending fate. This made me feel so empty.

Somehow, as I looked at the cows getting closer to the door of the killing floor of the slaughterhouse, it seemed apparent that they could sense their fate. I'm sure that they knew what was about to happen to them. Why else would they be so nervous—even mad? I'm certain that cows have more intelligence than we give them credit for having. Surely, if dogs can be trained to do tricks, killer whales to jump out of the water on command, bears to wrestle humans, rats to run a maze, monkeys to star in movies, etc., etc., then surely it should not seem too far-fetched to suppose that these animals can sense, perhaps even know when others in front of them are being killed and to know that the line of death ends in their own death. Clearly, at this point, the cows are stressed, their heart rate is increased as well as their respiratory rate, adrenaline, and cortisol, the stress hormone, is flowing through their bodies, and in this state, they are to be killed.

The line of death for the cows ended at a door at the rear of the slaughterhouse. The metal door was lifted, and here, one cow at a time, was led into a small-enclosed area similar to a concrete box with the top removed. The enclosed area was a little larger than the cow. Once inside this enclosed area, the door is shut immediately behind the cow. Now the cow could not move forward, backward, or to either side nor are they able to jump out of it. At this point, the poor cow was frantic and panic-stricken. It was breathing rapidly and looked really scared, as though it was about to cry. The same big, burly white man who shut the door behind the cow walked over to his station, which was right above the enclosed area. Here, he picked up a device called a stunner, which is actually a high-compression gun, and proceeded to load it. He took a quick look at the poor cow and started to place the gun on the cow's head. As he got closer to the cow, the cow made a considerable effort to escape. It tried to kick and jump, but to no avail. It had nowhere to go! The man placed the gun perfunctorily on the cow's head just above and between its eyes as its head was still for a split second and without the least showing of any emotion, pressed the trigger. BOOM!!! The sound the stun gun made was similar to that of a large caliber gun. The sound of the shot, along with the instantaneous cracking and penetration of the skull, was horrifying!!!

As soon as the gun discharged, the cow's eyes got big, as if they were about to blow out of their sockets! Then, there was the nauseating sound of that big 1,500-pound animal collapsing to the floor! My 1,500-pound pet of a few minutes was now lying on its side completely unconscious, drooling, and making random jerking movements. The high compression gun did not kill the cow but rendered it brain dead. The gun has a probe that is several inches long and contains a charge device. When the gun is pressed on the cow's head and fired, the probe penetrates the skull about five inches, and the charge renders the cow unconscious but keeps the heart beating.

The same man who fired the gun then flipped the large metal door, which made up one side of the enclosed area, an action that effectively forces the lifeless cow out of the enclosed area and into another area. The door was flipped again to enclose the area once again, making the area ready for the next cow. With his well-worn leather work gloves, he then grabbed heavy metal chains that were hanging from the overhead conveyor and placed them on one of the cow's hind legs. He then pulled on a chain, which hoisted the cow into the air with its hind leg stretched toward the ceiling. Being suspended in the air like this had to be painful, but since the cow was rendered brain dead, it is likely it did not feel any pain. With its head facing the floor, the cow began spewing out saliva, water, and the food that was left in its system.

The overhead conveyor moved the stunned cow to the next station, the "sticking" station. Here a middle-aged, neurotic-looking, skinny black man who appeared to be borderline emaciated, wearing a yellow rubber apron, steadied the twisting, writhing cow. With its heart still beating in its chest, the man took the longest and sharpest knife that I have ever seen in my life and proceeded to stab it into the cow's upper chest and began to cut down through the throat and toward the jaw, effectively severing its carotid arteries and jugular veins. SPLASH!!! Gallons of blood came rushing out of the cow like water from a pipe that burst. Blood flew out and went all over the man and his knife. The most frequently occurring abuse was in the horrific way cows were slaughtered.

Before the knife slices through a cow's throat, severing the carotid artery and jugular vein, the cows are supposed to be stunned with a bolt so that they are knocked unconscious and feel no pain. That is the theory anyway. That is not the reality. Often, the animal is not knocked out and rendered fully unconscious. Consequently, it feels the knife pierce its throat—the death stab. I could not believe my eyes! This was much worse than my experience in the butcher shop. Blood was everywhere; the floor was covered with blood. Words cannot describe the sight! It was no wonder that the man doing this was neurotic-looking. As he pulled the knife out of the cow, his hands, as well as the knife, were barely visible because of the flood of blood. The special effects of Hollywood could not approach this grotesque scene. Interestingly enough, this is supposed to be a humane way of killing! Just five minutes earlier, my "pet" was alive and begging for its life; now it was dead, murdered! For what??? To satisfy the carnal lusting for the luxury of meat—a burger, a steak.

I lost sight of Milton temporarily, but when I did spot him, he appeared to be just as in as much shock and horror as I was. I brought my faithful 35mm Nikon FM with me and was able to capture these horrors on film. The man who sliced the cow's throat saw me with the camera. He pointed the knife he used to kill the cow at me and told me in no uncertain terms not to photograph him. To this day, I think about that man and what his life must be like. I wonder if he has mental issues, nightmares, if he is ashamed of his job, gets angry at himself, and does he suffer from depression. How a man in such a position could function escapes me.

Next, the conveyor moved the carcass to the next station, where a healthy-looking black man made good use of powerful saws to cut off the lower parts of the legs. The noise that these saws made while they were cutting through the bones of the legs made me cringe! The smell of bone dust from the saws cutting through the legs was nauseating. The parts of the legs that were cut off were then tossed into a large barrel, making a flat thud sound as they landed on top of other shanks. Next, smaller chains were placed on the animal in several places. The chains were connected to a noisy machine. With the press of a button, the noisy machine began to pull the chains. I watched in disbelief as the chains pulled the entire hide off in one complete piece! The bloody hide was then dropped onto a bloody metal ramp and slid down into a container with other hides. These hides would likely be sold to a tannery and end up making everything from leather shoes to leather car seats.

Once the hide was removed, another worker came over like clockwork with a long knife. The man grabbed the cow's head and began to cut it off! I could not believe it! The head was then taken to another area of the slaughterhouse, where it was to be broken down into its component parts. Here the skin, tongue, brain, muscles of the mouth and cheek were removed and placed in their respective containers. It was placed on a machine that, at the touch of a button, cracks the skull open like a walnut. The brain is then removed, and the skull tossed into a large, unmarked container. To put it in the words of the owner of this slaughterhouse, "nothing is wasted."

As the carcass continued along on the conveyor, its tail was cut off, and various other procedures were performed. Now the carcass bore no resemblance to the 1,500-pound animal that I had just seen a few short minutes earlier. Its hide was gone; its shanks and head were also gone.

The areas where they once were now dripped with blood. I found it hard to believe that I was witnessing the automated, cold-blooded, wholesale murder of animals. Suddenly, I felt a fleeting fear for my own life. The reality of it all seemed like a horrible dream, a nightmare. I felt uneasy as I thought about how easy it would be for me to be dismembered. Who could tell my flesh from the cows?

The bloody carcass passed on to yet another station. Here a worker with yet another knife went up to the front of the carcass and began to cut from one end of it to the other. Immediately its innards came falling out onto a conveniently-placed cart. The stomachs, intestines, liver, pancreas, heart, kidneys all came right out. The worker then took the cart that contained the innards to another area of the slaughterhouse. Here the organs were separated and placed in their respective containers. The stomachs were cut open and their contents placed in another container.

The only thing that remained of my 1,500-pound friend was its sides. Now, these were wrapped and placed in a large refrigerator with numerous others. His journey was over. His short life of only one-and-a-half years had come to an abrupt, violent, heinous end. Sadness came over me. In the background noise, I could hear the sound of the gun being fired, signaling the beginning of the destruction of another innocent 1,500-pound cow. Soon, it too would be reduced to several hundred pounds of meat ranging from hamburger to prime rib. Why??? Why??? Why???

After our informal tour of the slaughterhouse, Milton and I were both left speechless and incredulous with what we saw, smelled, and heard. We resolved to come back again the next day for more photos. When we came back the next day, we were still welcomed with no strings attached. Since we knew what was in store for us, there were no surprises. However, the sounds now had meaning as we knew what was occurring. The sound of the stun gun in the background caused me to have flashbacks, and I found myself extremely uncomfortable, even on the verge of feeling sick being in the slaughterhouse. Milton must have felt the same way because we ended up cutting our visit short.

This happens every day across America. Millions of cattle are killed every year in the United States, and a significant number of those cows are dairy cows that are no longer productive, which is usually four to five years. Their normal lifespan is between fifteen to twenty years.

Can we continually kill, slaughter, and murder animals and eat their flesh without suffering any negative effects on our human nature?

The Meat-packing Industry—The Most Dangerous Occupation in the United States

There are approximately 150,000 workers in the meatpacking industry in the U.S. It is the most dangerous occupation. In any given year, one out of every four workers in this industry is injured, according to published data. In all likelihood, the rate of injury is much higher since there is great incentive not to report injuries. The injuries reported to the Occupational Safety and Health Administration range from the bizarre to the mundane. Workers' fingers, hands, and arms are amputated in a variety of machines. Workers are also killed on the job by chemical spills or machines going awry.

The risk of injury is ever-present due to the goal of keeping the "disassembly" line going. As many as 400 cattle pass by a station every hour. At such speeds, it is common for workers wielding knives to accidentally stab themselves or others nearby.

The low pay and terrible working conditions make it difficult to attract workers. Hence, only those who are incredibly desperate for employment tend to work in these horror-filled places. The jobs are often filled by migrant workers who are accustomed to making less in one day than they get paid for one hour's work in the meat-packing plant. This serves the industry fine since these workers are less likely to report an injury, join a union, complain about wages, or even file a lawsuit.

The situation is not likely to improve any time soon. Thirty years ago, the four largest meat packers controlled about 20 percent of the market. Today the same four companies control about 85 percent of the market. This gives these companies so much influence legally and politically, making it nearly impossible for change to occur.

Chapter 4

MEAT INSPECTION, AN IMPOSSIBLE TASK

In order for one to understand and appreciate the problems of the USDA in implementing its meat and poultry inspection program, one must consider the scale and extent of its operations. The Meat and Poultry Inspection Program has the arduous task of overseeing 6,200 meat, poultry, and other species establishments in the United States. These goings-on include, but are not limited to, the inspection of animals, inspection of sanitary conditions, and the prevention of false and deceptive labeling, as well as inspecting meat and meat products that come into the United States from practically every country in the world. In addition, this federal program employs only 3,500 inspectors to perform antemortem and postmortem inspections. These inspectors are civil servants, some of whom are graduates from veterinary college, while others are non-professional.

In June of 1906, the Meat Inspection Act was the official start of federal meat inspection in the United States. Prior to this time, there was no comprehensive, uniform, nationwide system of meat inspection. As a result, unfit animals undoubtedly ended up on the plates of many individuals. Unscrupulous individuals in the meat industry at that time were free to market unfit animals without the fear of penalty. The goals of the Meat Inspection Act were: 1) Detection and destruction of diseased and unfit meat: This included the condemnation of animal carcasses that were identified as not being fit for humans to consume, and that ultimately, were to be destroyed or used for fertilizer. It also included the retention of animal carcasses that were suspicious and yet could be passed as being fit for human consumption once all of the obvious abnormalities were removed. 2) The clean and sanitary handling and/or preparation of food that is completely or partly composed of meat. This is an extensive aspect of the act in that it means first that the construction of all plants must conform to the standards outlined by the USDA.

> In order for one to understand and appreciate the problems of the USDA in implementing its meat and poultry inspection program, one must consider the scale and extent of its operations.

It is also under this provision that inspectors oversee the practice of sanitary standards of handling products and sanitary standards of plant maintenance. 3) Prevention of harmful substances in meat food: This task is accomplished with the assistance of the USDA Food Safety and Inspection Service, which lists proprietary substances and non-food that are authorized for use under the USDA inspection and grading programs. 4) Application of an inspection mark. 5) Prevention of false or deceptive labeling or publication of misleading statements.

Perhaps the major problem regarding the implementation of its program is the vagueness of its goals. As an example, the detecting and the destroying of diseased and unfit meat are very broad. What constitutes "unfit meat"? To what extent is diseased meat "diseased"? As it stands, "unfit meat" can mean one thing to the federal government, another thing to the meat plant, another thing to the meat inspector, another thing to a pathologist, and yet another thing to the consumer. The same holds true for "diseased" meat. This boils down to a simple case of different actors with different perceptions. What one may consider to be a severe case of a dreaded disease may very well be considered as a disease by another as not being at all dangerous to the general public. Hence its presence to a small degree may not be at all alarming and may, in fact, be passed on as being "fit for human consumption."

In 1967, the Wholesome Meat Act was passed. Its original intent was to assure those who purchased meats in the United States that they would be able to purchase only wholesome, inspected, and approved meats. But unfortunately, once again, the vagueness of this act brought problems with its implementation. "Wholesome" can take on an entirely different meaning to the meat inspector, meat plant owner, the program director, etc. In the mind of the meat plant owner, an animal with cancerous organs is "wholesome" once the affected organs are removed. But certainly, this would not be so in the minds of most consumers!!!

There is a great deal of inconsistency in policy direction regarding what the meat plant owners determine as being "wholesome" and "fit for human consumption" and what the federal and state programs determine to be "wholesome" and "fit for human consumption." Individual states were able to become directly involved in meat inspection under the Talmadge-Aiken Act. Under this act the federal government shares the costs of inspection with the states. Hence, states with a large cattle and poultry industry, such as California and Texas, have powerful lobbies and influence with respect to manipulating legislation on the state and federal levels.

One of the more frustrating tasks in writing this book is the degree to which government is no longer transparent. Today, meat inspection is under the USDA's Food Safety Inspection Service. The following information is from the now defunct FSIS website: http://www.fsis.usda.gov/Fact_Sheets/Slaughter_Inspection_101/index.asp. This website has been replaced with this new website: **https://1ref.us/1y9** (accessed June 2, 2022). The old website was far more explicit in detailing the inspection process which the new website lacks. Was this on purpose???

About The Food Safety and Inspection Service

USDA's Food Safety and Inspection Service (FSIS) is responsible for ensuring the safety and wholesomeness of meat, poultry, and processed egg products and ensuring that it is accurately labeled.

FSIS enforces the Federal Meat Inspection Act (FMIA), the Poultry Products Inspection Act (PPIA), and the Egg Products Inspection Act. These laws require Federal inspection and regulation of meat, poultry, and processed egg products prepared for distribution in commerce for use as human food. It also verifies compliance with the Humane Methods of Slaughter Act for livestock. This statute is enforced through the FMIA,

FSIS employs about 7,800 in-plant inspection program personnel. They inspect more than 6,200 federally inspected establishments. These establishments vary greatly in size and type of activity conducted.

Inspection Basics

Industry is accountable for producing safe food. Whereas Government is responsible for: Conducting carcass by carcass inspection, setting appropriate food safety standards, verifying through inspection that those standards are met, and maintaining a strong enforcement program to deal with plants that do not meet regulatory standards.

Slaughter facilities cannot conduct slaughter operations if FSIS inspection personnel are not present. Only federally inspected establishments can produce products that are destined to enter interstate commerce or for export to foreign countries. To receive Federal inspection, an establishment must apply for and receive an official Grant of Inspection. To obtain this, an establishment must: Have written Sanitation Standard Operating Procedures; Conduct a hazard analysis; Develop and validate a Hazard Analysis and Critical Control Point (HACCP) Plan; and agree to abide by all FSIS regulations.

FSIS conducts carcass-by-carcass inspection at all federally inspected slaughter facilities and verifies that establishments follow all food safety and humane handling regulations. FSIS inspection program personnel verify that the establishment maintains proper sanitation procedures; it follows its HACCP plan and complies with all FSIS regulations pertaining to slaughter and processing operations. If the establishment fails to maintain sanitation, does not follow its HACCP plan, or violates other regulations, FSIS inspection program personnel will issue a citation to the establishment in the form of a noncompliance record to document the noncompliance. If necessary, they could also take regulatory control action.

Livestock slaughter and processing establishments must maintain written procedures for removing, segregating, and disposing of specified risk materials (SRMs) so they do not enter the food supply. SRMs are high-risk tissues that pose the greatest risk of containing the agent associated with bovine spongiform encephalopathy (also known as BSE or "mad cow disease"). Some examples of SRMs are the brain, skull, eyes, trigeminal ganglia, spinal cord, vertebral column, and dorsal root ganglia of cattle thirty months of age and older; the tonsils of all cattle; and the distal ileum of all cattle.

The causative agent of BSE, prions, is not limited to the locations identified as SRMs. Virtually every part of the animal is SRM because it can be found in the blood, and blood flows to virtually every part of the animal. To think that SRM is the answer is to engage in a form of prevention that does nothing more than give the illusion of security.

Inspection Process

Antemortem (before slaughter)

Establishments are required to notify FSIS inspection program personnel when they want animals inspected prior to slaughter. Inspection at a slaughter establishment begins in the antemortem area or pen where FSIS inspection program personnel inspect live animals before, in motion, and at rest on the day of slaughter. If the animal is acceptable, it is passed for slaughter. If the animal is not acceptable, it will be cast into one of several categories:

1. U.S. Suspect: these animals are generally seriously crippled, test positive for TB, are immature, or have a "minor" epithelioma (cancer) of the eye or orbital region.
2. U.S. Condemned: these are animals that are "downers," about to die, comatose, have fevers, die in the pen, or have obvious symptoms of disease.
3. FSIS 5-04 Notice: these are non-ambulatory disabled cattle. A veterinarian medical officer will condemn these animals as well as all cattle showing central nervous system symptoms regardless of ability to ambulate.
4. If not already dead, condemned animals are killed by the establishment and cannot enter the establishment to be slaughtered or dressed.

It is the establishment's responsibility to follow the Humane Methods of Slaughter Act. Egregious violations of humane handling requirements can lead to suspension of inspection activity within an establishment. This will stop the plant from operating.

Noncompliance records for humane handling also can be issued when the violation is less than egregious, such as not having water available in pens. During this inspection, FSIS inspection program personnel observe all animals at rest and in motion. Inspection program personnel are trained to look for abnormalities and signs that could indicate disease or health conditions that would prohibit the animal from entering the food supply. If an animal goes down or shows signs of illness after receiving and passing antemortem inspection before slaughter, the establishment must immediately notify the FSIS veterinarian to make a case-by-case disposition of the animal's condition.

Alternatively, the establishment may humanely euthanize the animal. These animals are labeled as "U.S. Suspect" and are segregated until the animal has received additional inspection by an FSIS veterinarian. FSIS veterinarians and other inspection personnel are not stationed in the antemortem area for the entire day. They do return randomly to verify humane handling, as well as the stunning and bleeding process.

Other inspection activities are also conducted off-line inside the slaughter facility when antemortem inspections have been completed. These off-line FSIS inspection program personnel move through the different areas of the establishment while performing their duties. This gives them the ability to vary their assigned off-line inspections.

According to the Animal Disposition Reporting System (ADRS), which is a subunit of the Food Safety and Inspection Service (FSIS), which is a subunit of the United States Department of Agriculture (USDA), the following conditions result in antemortem condemnation of cattle: emaciation, miscellaneous degenerative and dropsic conditions, actinomycosis, actinobacil, TB rector and no-reactor, arthritis, eosinophilic myositis, mastitis, metritis, nephritis pyelitis, pericarditis, peritonitis, pneumonia, uremia, carcinoma, epithelioma, malignant lymphoma, sarcoma, misc. neoplasms, cysticercosis, myiasis, toxemia, miscellaneous parasitic conditions, abscess pyemia, septicemia, contamination, and icterus. Of the above-mentioned conditions, more cattle are condemned antemortem for lymphoma and pneumonia than anything else.

Postmortem or after slaughter

Postmortem inspection occurs in the slaughter area after the animal has been humanely stunned and bled. FSIS inspection program personnel perform carcass-by-carcass postmortem inspections. Agency inspection personnel are stationed at fixed positions along the slaughter line and are known as on-line inspectors. Inspectors look for signs of disease or pathological conditions that would render a carcass or part unwholesome or otherwise unfit for human consumption. Any carcass in need of further diagnosis or disposition is segregated, and the veterinarian summoned.

In a feeble attempt to minimize the spread of "Mad Cow" disease, SRM material is removed from cattle. For cattle thirty months of age or older, this includes the brain, skull, eyes, trigeminal, ganglia, spinal cord, most of the vertebral column, and the dorsal root ganglia. For all cattle it includes the tonsils and the distal ileum of the small intestine.

The establishment must maintain the identity of every carcass and ensure that the retained carcasses do not enter the food supply until FSIS inspection program personnel release it. After further inspection, if a carcass has no generalized signs of disease or pathological conditions, it is passed without restriction and may enter the food supply. Localized conditions are removed prior to the carcass entering the food supply.

What happens to the condemned animals and parts? The carcass may be used for food after the affected parts are removed and the remainder cooked or frozen. Condemned animals supposedly do not enter the food chain. However, they enter the human food chain by the "back door" via:

1.   Rendering – made into inedible fats, greases, or oils
2.   Tanked – made into animal feed or fertilizer
3.   Frozen – held at 10ºF for five days and then sold as animal feed.

Off-line FSIS inspection program personnel also observe the sanitary conditions of those parts of the slaughter area not directly related to carcass inspection, such as where the hides are removed.

A major problem of implementation of the meat inspection program is that of consensual imperative. Its presence in the Meat and Poultry Inspection Program is evidenced by the many interest groups that lobbied successfully to increase the amount of fillers used to stretch various meat products. The more common fillers are blood and bonemeal. By increasing the amount of fillers, especially blood, in meat products, there is an increase in the likelihood of these products being unfit for human consumption. This is likely to result due to the multitude of disease-causing organisms that are in blood. The problem is exacerbated further when blood, bone meal, and other fillers originate from condemned carcasses and carcasses that have been retained due to suspicion of any number of anomalies.

Another example of the immense power with which the meat industry can control government and get its way is the number of birds allowed to be inspected per minute. During the time President Carter was in office, the number of birds inspected per minute went from forty-five to seventy. A short time later, under the Reagan administration, the number was raised again from seventy to eighty-five. By almost doubling their rate of birds per minute, those with a personal stake in the meat industry have guaranteed themselves a hefty profit with little, if any, increase in costs for them. The sad part of the story is that such an action increases considerably the chances of diseased animals ending up as food in the marketplace.

One factor which is responsible for the failure of programs during implementation is the inadequate scope of effort. The task that the Meat and Poultry Inspection program has set out to accomplish is grandiose given its limited resources. Because of the vast scope of the task, in order for the Meat and Poultry Inspection Program to be successful, it must coordinate efforts with other programs that are out of its control. The Meat and Poultry Inspection program has no direct control over the use of pesticides, herbicides, insecticides, growth hormones, and other chemicals used in the production of meat. Without the coordination and cooperation of the various agencies, departments, and farmers, the Meat and Poultry Inspection Program will be frustrated in its attempt to provide meat products that are "wholesome" and "fit for human consumption."

The inadequate scope of effort is also evident by the poor resource allocation of the Meat and Poultry Inspection Program. There are approximately only 3,500 inspectors employed by the USDA to inspect animals. Their job is to examine each carcass and check for evidence of diseases and other gross abnormalities and conditions. This sounds simple enough on the surface, but when one digs a little deeper, one will be surprised at the overwhelming task meat inspectors have. The particular slaughterhouse that Milton and I visited murdered on an average day 250 cattle during a regular eight-hour day. Just prior to the major holidays, when the demand for beef is higher, they can boost the number of murders to 350 per eight-hour workday, which would be just about their maximum capacity. Simple mathematics will show us that in an average eight-hour workday, when 250 cattle are killed, that translates into thirty-one cattle killed each hour. Furthermore, on a heavy day when the slaughterhouse is working at or near its maximum capacity of killing 350 cattle per eight-hour day, forty-four cattle must be killed each hour. This means that the one federal meat inspector at this particular slaughterhouse has the gruesome task of having to inspect anywhere between 250–350 dead cattle in just eight hours each working day! That roughly calculates to a grand total of about anywhere from 1.3–2 minutes to inspect each mercilessly murdered cow!

There are much larger slaughterhouses owned by large corporations that murder in excess of 3,000 cattle in an average eight-hour day! Imagine how the meat inspectors in those plants feel! The situation is even more ridiculous in slaughterhouses that kill smaller animals, such as pigs and chickens. In large, automated slaughterhouses such as these, thousands upon thousands are killed each day and subsequently must be inspected. In such situations, the inspectors have literally just a few short seconds to inspect the animal carcass as it comes to a brief stop at his/her inspection station.

In these few short seconds, the meat inspector is expected to be able to examine the dead animal, check all of its parts, organs, and body tissues for evidence of diseases, parasitic infections, and other abnormal conditions that would render it unsafe or unfit for human consumption as food. Impossible!!!!! For example, in 1960, 26 million cattle were killed for food in the United States. Of these, 75 percent were under federal inspection. In 1982, 36.2 million cattle were killed, and 95 percent of these were under federal inspection. Furthermore, in 1960, a total of 135,000,000 cattle, calves, sheep, goats, pigs, and horses were slaughtered in the United States. Of these, 78 percent were under federal inspection. In 1982, 128,800,000 cattle, calves, sheep, pigs, goats, and horses were slaughtered and of these, 95 percent were under federal inspection. In 1982, 3,195,000 calves, 5,464,000 sheep and lambs, 22,882,000 ducks, 35,913,000 cattle, 77,290,000 hogs, 196,000,000 turkeys, and 4,833,665,000 chickens, making a grand total of 5,174,409,000 animals were federally inspected. Even more astounding is the fact that the number of animals killed per year continues to rise. In 2020, 32,886,000 cattle, 2,225,400 calves, 131,639,900 hogs, 3,556,000 sheep and lambs, 224,000,000 turkeys, and 9,408,934,900 chickens were federally inspected and slaughtered for food. That is a staggering 8,692,497,000 carcasses federally inspected! If the 3,500 meat inspectors worked a forty-hour work week all year without vacation, sick leave, lunch breaks, etc., they would have an average time of only five seconds to inspect each carcass!

Animals are inspected before and after slaughter. Animals with the most blatant signs of disease may be condemned. The carcasses may

> *In these few short seconds, the meat inspector is expected to be able to examine the dead animal, check all of its parts, organs, and body tissues for evidence of diseases, parasitic infections, and other abnormal conditions that would render it unsafe or unfit for human consumption as food.*

be used for food after the affected parts are removed and the remainder cooked or frozen. Meat inspectors condemn a seemingly considerable number of animals each year. Given the overwhelming demands placed on meat inspectors, the number of animals condemned is only a fraction of the number that should be condemned and represent the animals that were the sickest and showed the most blatant signs of disease. Bear in mind that there are a number of diseases that are not cause for condemnation, BLV and BIV chief among them. Furthermore, there is not a way to detect Mad Cow disease in cattle that are not showing any symptoms!

Given the burden placed on meat inspectors, it is quite obvious that there is a lot of underreporting. In 1990 (the last year these figures were easily made available to the public), 33,033,653 cattle were inspected, and only 149,999 (less than 0.46 percent) were condemned. It would appear that the overwhelming majority of cattle are healthy. However, when you consider that 6,584,975 (20 percent) of the cattle inspected had their liver condemned, it is apparent that there are many more sick animals than the number actually condemned, and, of course, these animals end up as food for the consumer. 1990 was the last year that the government made these statistics available. Perhaps they did not want to frighten the general meat-eating public! Perhaps even more disturbing is the number of carcasses retained for various diseases then subsequently passed for food after the affected parts are removed and the number of carcasses passed for food after "processing."

Fortunately, the inspection process does not stop here. The billions of carcasses of animals are turned into meat. In 2020, over 85,000,000,000 pounds of meat and poultry were federally inspected.1 In addition, another 14,000,000,000 pounds of meat and poultry were imported into the U.S. that were also federally inspected.2 Meat products are inspected during and after processing. The problem is that by the time one of the foregoing conditions is discovered, the product has often already made its way into the grocery stores, restaurants, and even to the stomachs of consumers!

What Happens to Tainted Meat?

According to statistics furnished by the Food Safety and Inspection Service of the U.S. Department of Agriculture, millions upon millions of pounds of meat have been recalled. Some of the major reasons for the recall centered around meat that was under-processed, Salmonella,

Listeria, and E. coli. When these conditions are discovered, the products involved are immediately recalled.

The largest meat recall in history took place in 2008. A disquieting 143,400,000 pounds of beef were recalled.3 By the time the recall had taken place, the UDSA was of the belief that most of the beef had already been eaten. The slaughterhouse in question was shut down because it slaughtered "downer" cattle, those too sick to be able to walk on their own. Many of these cattle may have been suffering from Mad Cow disease since the inability to stand alone is one of the distinguishing characteristics of the disease. The startling fact is less than 1.4 percent of the beef had been recovered! The year 2019 was a busy year for meat recalls. There were 131 meat recalls that year that involved millions of pounds of meat. The paltry amount of meat that is recovered shows the inability as well as the impossibility of the inspection process to protect the consumer.

What happens to the rest of the tainted meat that is not recovered? It can end up in pet food, in school lunches, restaurants, grocery stores, or even on your plate!

Meat inspection is an impossible task!

Chapter 5

OH CRAP!

The Yellow and Brown
the Green Movement Ignores!

Cows are often shown on many milk cartons, billboards, and magazine ads grazing on a pasture next to a country barn. This is the way it was years ago when cows had plenty of room to roam and forage. The urine and manure these animals generated was not a problem since it was often used as fertilizer for crops on the farm or a local farm to grow crops that were then fed to the animals. For instance, in 1940, there were 4,663,431 dairies dotted across the United States. The average number of dairy cows on these dairy farms was five![58]

Today, the reality is quite different from that pictured in the media and milk cartons. Today, there are only 34,187 dairies in the U.S., with an average of 273 cows per dairy. Increasingly, milk is coming from animal feeding operations (AFO) and confined animal feeding operations (CAFOs). AFOs concentrate animals, feed, manure and urine, dead animals, and production operations all in one place. Instead of the animals grazing naturally, the feed is brought to the animals. There are approximately 450,000 AFOs in the United States.[59]

CAFOs are AFOs with a minimum of 1,000 animal units. An animal unit is an animal equivalent of 1,000 pounds live weight and equates to 1,000 head of beef cattle, 700 dairy cows, 2,500 swine weighing more than 55 lbs., 125,000 broiler chickens, or 82,000 laying hens or pullets confined on site for more than forty-five days during the year. Any AFO

---

58 Don P. Blayney, "The Changing Landscape of U.S. Milk Production," USDA Statistical Bulletin Number 978 (June 2002): 2, https://1ref.us/1x6 (accessed https://1ref.us/1x6).
59 "Animal Feeding Operations," USDA Natural Resources Conservation Service, https://1ref.us/1ya (accessed June 2, 2022).

that discharges manure or wastewater into a natural or man-made ditch, stream, or other waterway is defined as a CAFO, regardless of size.[60] There are more than 20,000 CAFOs in the U.S.[61]

A milking dairy cow consumes between thirty to fifty gallons of water and consumes 110 to 170 pounds of wet feed each day.[62] Since what goes in must come out, a dairy cow excretes 120 pounds of manure and about three gallons of urine each day.[63] Do you understand these numbers and what they mean? It takes 4.3 to 5.1 gallons of water and 13.8 to 21.3 pounds of feed to produce one, just one, gallon of milk! With respect to resources, this is udder insanity!!!

In addition, fifteen pounds of manure are generated for every gallon of milk that is produced. That means that in the liberal, environmentally-conscious state of California, its 1,725,000 dairy cows, on average, will consume 69,000,000 gallons of water, 241,500,000 pounds of feed, produce 207,000,000 pounds of manure, and 5,175,000 gallons of urine each and every day of the week just to produce 13,800,000 gallons of milk containing 10,707,765,000,000,000 somatic cells!

In a given year, the dairy cows in the Golden State will consume 25,185,000,000, yes, more than 25 BILLION gallons of water; 88,147,500,000, yes, more than 88 BILLION pounds of feed! These same Golden State cows will produce 75,555,000,000, yes, more than 75 BILLION pounds of manure, and 1,888,875,000, yes, nearly 2 BILLION gallons of urine, just to produce 5,037,000,000 gallons of milk with 3,908,334,200,000,000,000 somatic cells!!!

To help you get a better perspective on how much water dairy cattle in California consume, I will use the largest oil supertanker; it holds 84,000,000 gallons of oil and is more than a quarter of a mile in length. The amount of water that dairy cows consume per year would require 300 of these supertankers! If they were arranged in a straight line, they would stretch for more than eighty-five miles, the distance from San Francisco to Sacramento!

---

60 "Animal Feeding Operations."
61 Christopher Walljasper, "Large Animal Feeding Operations on the Rise," June 7, 2018, https://1ref.us/1yb (accessed June 2, 2022).
62 Craig Thomas, "Drinking Water for Dairy Cattle: Part 1," Michigan State University Extension, April 5, 2011, https://1ref.us/1yc (accessed June 2, 2022).
63 Thomas, "Drinking Water—Part 1."

Now, let's look at what is involved on a national scale to produce milk. There are approximately 9,340,000 dairy cattle in the United States. In one year, these cows will consume 136,364,000,000 gallons of water and 477,274,000,000 pounds of wet feed. They will produce 409,092,000,000 pounds of manure and 10,227,300,000 gallons of urine all to make 27,272,800,000 gallons of milk that will contain at least 19,303,551,000,000,000,000 somatic (pus) cells!

The amount of drinking water that dairy cows consume each year in the U.S. is unsustainable. Moreover, there is a worldwide shortage of clean drinkable water. Using our supertanker illustration again, it would require 1,623 supertankers filled to capacity with water to equal the amount of water dairy cattle consume each year in the U.S. If placed in a straight line, these tankers would stretch 462 miles, the distance from New York to Cleveland, OH!!!

Let me attempt to make these numbers even more understandable and to show their significance. The amount of water dairy cattle consume each year in the U.S. is enough to give every human being living in the world one gallon of water every day for more than two weeks! It is enough to give every person in the U.S., including those who are in the country illegally, a gallon of water each day for more than a year! It is enough water to give everyone living in Houston and Atlanta one gallon a day for ten years! Lest I be remiss and not include golf lovers, it is enough water to water every golf course in California, Arizona, South Carolina, North Carolina, and Florida combined for an entire year. These figures do not include the amount of water that goes into growing the feed and washing down the waste these animals produce. If those figures were included, the above numbers would certainly more than double!!!

However, as wasteful as milk is, ice cream and cheese are even more wasteful. You may ask yourself, "How can that be?" It takes approximately eight gallons of milk to make one gallon of ice cream! It takes ten pounds of milk to make one pound of cheese! How can we justify such wasteful use of water? We cannot! It is udder insanity to do so.

Now, let us look at all of the manure that dairy cattle generate. Where does all of this crap go? Where can you put 409,092,000,000 pounds of manure? To conceptualize how much crap this crap really is, if one were to fill the fifty-three-foot trailers that semi-trucks pull down the highway with the manure that is generated in one year from dairy cows, it would require 5,113,650 of them. If placed in a line, they would form a line long enough to be able to go around the world not once but twice! This is more than one and a half times the total amount of all of the fecal matter produced by every man, woman, and child in the United States—Udder insanity!!!

This monumental amount of manure, along with urine, is stored in lagoons and sprayed on surrounding property. This is problematic for several reasons. One reason is that this manure is loaded with nitrogen and phosphorus. By spraying this mixture of urine and feces into the air, these chemicals become airborne and can travel for miles. There have been a number of reports of people living near these vast lagoons who have suffered respiratory problems as a result of the spraying.

The lagoons that hold all of this manure and urine are not always lined, so as a consequence, they are subject to leaking. As the effluent leaks, it will eventually make its way into the underlying water aquifers. This can result in water having high levels of nitrates and other chemicals, thereby making the water from wells unfit for human consumption. These lagoons also run the risk of overflowing and breaching, leading to the spillage of untold millions of gallons that can find its way into streams and estuaries. For example, North Carolina recently renewed its ban on any new hog CAFOs after 25 million gallons of hog waste spilled into the New River. When either breach or overflow occurs, the runoff can result in the pollution of waterways and eventually find itself in nearby lakes, rivers, and the ocean. Such contamination leads to an increase in nitrate levels and a host of microorganisms. When the waterways become contaminated with the runoff, the oxygen in the water is taken up by the waste, thereby making less oxygen available to fish and other creatures that live in the water. This can result in the death of untold numbers of fish and creatures that inhabit the waterways. Conversely, when it is hot and dry, as the animal waste breaks down, it forms methane and ammonia. This, coupled with the dust that is generated, is a recipe for respiratory problems for people in the immediate area. As you can imagine, there are not enough lagoons to hold that much manure and urine.

> North Carolina recently renewed its ban on any new hog CAFOs after 25 million gallons of hog waste spilled into the New River.

Just as there is a concentration of dairy farms, there is a concentration of wealth and ownership that forces the small- and medium-sized operations out of business. Farm policies have more and more favored large operations rather than smaller ones. The larger operations can afford to lobby state legislators and Congress to enact legislation to favor them, whereas the smaller operations do not have that luxury and power. One way this is seen is in the relatively inexpensive cost of grain for feed. Grain is the largest expense of producing milk. Governments have enacted policies that allow for the production of inexpensive grain, which, of course, is of great benefit to the dairy farmer. The federal Farm Bill has been a consistent source of enacting policies that allow grain prices to decrease to such a low level, often lower than the cost of production. This is only viable by agricultural welfare in the form of subsidies to the grain farmers in the amounts of billions of dollars each year.[64]

It does not take a neurosurgeon to realize that the cost of producing milk is high, unprofitable, and incredibly wasteful. Each gallon of milk that is produced by the dairy farmer is done so at a loss. Many dairy farmers are trying to hold on in hopes that the price they get paid per gallon of milk will increase to a level that will be profitable. That is not likely to happen any time soon, given the marketplace, demand, and supply. It is only a matter of time before the dairy farmer goes into oblivion like the television repairman.

When Arnold Schwarzenegger was running for governor of the state of California, one of his major contributors to his campaign was Chuck Ahlem. Chuck was also a major contributor to the former governor, Gray Davis. Chuck is the founder of the world's largest single site-cheese and whey products manufacturing facility, the Hilmar Cheese Company. Ahlem also owns Ahlem Ranch, home to 1,700 dairy cows. His family also owns the ranch next door, home to an additional 3,700 milking cows.

How was good ol' Chucky rewarded for his contributions, a measly $21,200 to Arnold?[65] For starters, Chucky was appointed as the agriculture undersecretary for the state. For years, California water-quality enforcers have turned a blind eye toward the world's largest cheese factory, Hilmar Cheese, by sparing the company millions of dollars in required sewage treatment and allowing it to foul local water supplies and the air of nearby neighborhoods.

Hilmar Cheese Co. makes over a million pounds of cheese per day. Daily, Hilmar dumps an average of 1.5 MILLION gallons of wastewater.

64 "Subsidies," EWG, https://1ref.us/1yd (accessed June 2, 2022).
65 Bay Area New Group, "Hard Cheese: Factory Fined for Fouling Air, Water," *East Bay Times,* January 30, 2005, https://1ref.us/1ye (accessed June 2, 2022).

It was fined $4 million for violating wastewater standards by flushing fields with "cow water," a practice it had been doing for decades. The wastewater's volume and salinity have far exceeded limits imposed by the state's Central Valley Regional Water Quality Control Board to keep the groundwater drinkable for neighbors. The water board has recorded at least 4,000 violations against Hilmar Cheese from 2000 to 2004. Hilmar Cheese is one of California's largest and most chronic offenders of clean-water laws.

Historically, rather than fine or issue an injunction against Hilmar, the Valley water board raised the limit on wastewater volume, not surprisingly when the cheesemaker's production kept increasing. Board records show regulators agreed to increases four times in eight years—1990 through 1997—each time counting on company promises to cut pollution. Given all of the water that dairy cows consume and all of the groundwater, rivers, lakes, and streams that are polluted as a result of the poor disposal of the urine and feces these animals produce, where is the outrage and concern for the earth from the environmentalists, from the "Green" movement, from the Sierra Club, and from the Nobel Prize-winning Al Gore and his ilk? Surely, they are not ignorant of these facts? Why are they silent on these issues? Perhaps it is too much of an inconvenient truth for even Al Gore and others who claim to be so concerned about the earth to ponder as they gulp down milkshakes while eating cheeseburgers and pizza. Could it be that this inconvenient truth is too inconvenient? Could it be that since there is no way to make billions of dollars selling carbon credits by campaigning against the wastefulness of the dairy industry that it is better left alone? Could it be that maintaining the trappings of celebrity is more important than fighting against polluting groundwater? It seems that for Al Gore and his ilk, it is easier to be seen promoting carbon credits than truly saving the planet and making certain the inhabitants of the world have safe water to drink.

Daily we are made aware of the plight of those in the world who go to bed hungry every night because they do not have enough food to eat, yet we willingly ignore the nearly three billion pounds of feed given each year to dairy cows in the U.S. alone. There is so much talk about climate change and carbon footprints, but virtually no discussion about the mountains of feces you can step your foot in!

Finally, eliminating milk from the diet would do more than any single factor to reduce greenhouse gases, save fuel, save water, and eliminate world hunger. Consider the amount of fuel used to: 1) grow the enormous amounts of corn, grain, and soybeans (note the machines required for tilling, irrigation, crop dusting, etc.) that will be used for feed; 2) transport the grain and soybeans to manufacturers of feed on gas-guzzling, polluting big rigs; 3) operate the feed mills; 4) transport feed to the dairies; 5) operate the dairies; 6) operate the slaughterhouse; 7) transport the meat to processing plants; 8) operate the milk-processing plants; 9) transport the milk to grocery stores; 10) keep the milk refrigerated in the stores, until it's sold; 11) after they are used up and milked to death, truck the animals many miles to slaughter. Every single stage involves heavy pollution, massive amounts of greenhouse gases, and massive amounts of energy, yet there is silence on the subject. We are duped into thinking that not driving an SUV and recycling will save the planet ... THAT is the real CRAP of the Green Movement farce.

Chapter 6

GOT PROTEIN? WHAT DOESN'T???

Protein, protein, protein. Just what is protein? Well, the word *protein* originates from the Greek word *protos*, which means foremost or ahead of all others. Proteins can be found in every single cell in your body!

Proteins contain carbon, nitrogen, hydrogen, and oxygen, and some also contain sulfur and phosphorus. Proteins are composed of amino acids. The amino acids are linked together in a chain by peptide bonds to form protein. To be considered a protein, the chain must have at least fifty amino acids. Most proteins have well over fifty amino acids, and others may have over 1,000 amino acids.

The discovery of proteins is credited to Gerrit Mulder, who determined the elemental composition of several proteins, noting that they had a single common core. It was Jacob Berzelius who coined the term protein. Proteins play many key roles in the body. Proteins are the building blocks of the body as they are responsible for building and repairing tissues. They also function as hormones, regulating growth and development. Proteins function as enzymes, increasing the rates of chemical reactions. Proteins also function as antibodies. Antibodies are substances that seek out and destroy viruses, bacteria, and foreign substances. Muscles are made up of protein and, of course, are instrumental in movement. Your skin, hair, and nails are composed of protein. Hemoglobin is composed of protein. Hemoglobin is the part of the red blood cell that carries oxygen.

The need for protein is obvious and inescapable. There has been a push to have Americans consume protein. There has even been a bigger push to capitalize on the need for protein by certain industries.

Milk to the Rescue!

Our society is inundated with propaganda from the meat and dairy industry regarding the need for protein. Television, radio, and print media bombard the public with commercials advertising meat and milk in an all too successful attempt to perpetuate and condition us to believe that meat and milk are the answer to our protein needs. One print ad was even so cunning as to show a pregnant woman drinking a glass of milk, suggesting the use of milk gives the mother and her unborn child sufficient protein. The subtle message being that milk is what gives you protein and that milk is good for pregnant women and unborn children. This mass media protein blitz has created a condition in most of us that I call "hypoproteinaphobia"—simply the irrational fear of not getting enough protein in the diet.

Since we have been taught that milk has a lot of protein, our neurotic condition of "hypoproteinaphobia" pushes us to drink milk in order to acquire the protein we've been led to believe that we need. In effect, the little computer in our minds has been programmed to reason like this: I need protein, milk has protein, and therefore, I need to drink milk in order to get the protein that my body needs. Consequently, people everywhere buy milk for the sake of getting the protein they think they need. This conditioned reasoning and subsequent action is exploited by those with a personal stake in the dairy industry. This method alone is responsible for pumping billions of dollars into the dairy industry every year.

The dairy industry receives great assistance in their annual quest for billions of dollars from the ignorance of medical doctors. Most doctors have an extremely limited knowledge of nutrition. They have horrible health practices themselves and are often oblivious of the relationship between diet and health. This should not come as a complete surprise. Doctors are trained to diagnose illnesses, not how to prevent them. They are accustomed and trained to prescribe drugs rather than discuss with you changes that can be made in your lifestyle to better your health.

Those with a vested interest in the dairy industry would lead you to believe that if you don't drink milk, you will readily become protein deficient. Often cases are made in favor of "adequate" protein by showing malnourished people suffering from a host of health problems in an attempt to make you think that their condition is due to the result of a lack of protein. What they aren't telling you is that the people are suffering from a condition known as abrosia. Abrosia is simply the <u>lack of food</u>! Mothers suffering from abrosia will, of course, give birth to children suffering from malnutrition, which may very well manifest itself in a condition known as marasmus, a type of protein-calorie malnutrition. As a consequence, it should not come as a complete surprise that people who are grossly undernourished, who have not eaten a meal in weeks, would have a deficiency of virtually every mineral, vitamin as well as protein. It is the <u>lack of food</u> that is responsible for their health problems. Kwashiorkor was another alleged protein deficiency. However, it too has been dismissed as the person who named it saw it as a health fiction.

Children require protein primarily for growth, whereas adults require protein primarily for tissue repair. We lose less than an ounce of protein a day in our feces, urine, skin, hair, and perspiration! Consequently, contrary to popular opinion, it is easy to have "adequate" protein in the diet without having even a hint of meat. About the only way a person could not get "adequate" protein is to stop eating! Even the person with the poorest eating habits will have more than enough protein in their diet.

In order to have a true protein deficiency, one must plan carefully. The ideal candidate for this would be an abnormally thin pregnant woman. To make her deficient of protein, her diet would have to consist of nothing but pure water and rock candy, the type of candy that is made almost completely of sugar. It is a bit extreme, but that is the extent to which one must go in order to have protein deficiency. All plants and animals are composed of protein. Therefore, again, if one simply eats food, it is highly unlikely that one will develop a protein deficiency.

Foods are composed of fats, protein, and carbohydrates, all of which contain calories. "Complete" protein is composed of twenty different amino acids. Humans can produce ten of the twenty amino acids. It is claimed that the others must be obtained from the diet. However, the body is far more creative than many want to give credit for. We have been duped by the experts into believing that failure to obtain enough of even one of the ten essential amino acids, those that we cannot make, results in degradation of the body's proteins—muscle and so forth—to obtain the one amino acid that is needed.

It is extremely unlikely to find anyone, anywhere, with an amino acid deficiency. Unlike fat and starch, the human body does not store excess amino acids for later use—the amino acids must be in the food every day. However, if one does not acquire sufficient essential amino acids in the diet, all is not lost. The body can recycle proteins that it already has. This is achieved in the intestine. Each day, ninety grams of protein flow through the digestive tract, largely due to its constant rebuilding.[66] These proteins can be broken down as necessary into their individual amino acids to be used by the body as the body sees fit.

There is an issue in science regarding what and how many amino acids are "essential," that is, not produced by the body. For the sake of discussion, I will hold the number to ten. The ten amino acids that we can produce are alanine, asparagine, aspartic acid, cysteine, glutamic acid, glutamine, glycine, proline, serine, and tyrosine. Tyrosine is produced from phenylalanine, so if the diet is deficient in phenylalanine, tyrosine will be required as well. The essential amino acids are arginine (required for the young, but not for adults), histidine, isoleucine, leucine, lysine, methionine, phenylalanine, threonine, tryptophan, and valine. These amino acids are required in the diet. Why they are called "essential" is unclear because all the amino acids are "essential." Plants, of course, must be able to make all the amino acids. Humans, on the other hand, do not have all the enzymes required for the biosynthesis of all of the amino acids.

We are led to believe that the best way to get these "essential" amino acids in our diet is to eat meat and dairy products. Who has been convincing us of this for decades? You guessed it, the meat and dairy industry! We have been sold the lie that only the flesh of animals can provide all of the amino acids that the human body requires. Cow's milk is 87 percent water, which contains an average of 13 percent total solids and about 9 percent solids-not-fat. The total protein content of cow's milk is approximately 3.5 percent by weight (36 g/L), providing almost 38 percent of the total solids-not-fat content of milk, and about 21 percent of whole milk energy.

Milk proteins are divided into two major types: casein and whey. Casein constitutes approximately 80 percent (29.5 g/L) of the total protein in cow's milk, and whey protein accounts for about 20 percent (6.3 g/L).[67] It has four major types, including alpha- (αs1- and αs2-casein), beta-, gamma-, and kappa-casein.

66 D. Dallas et al., "Personalizing Protein Nourishment," *Critical Reviews in Food Science and Nutrition* 57, no. 15 (October 13, 2017): 3313–3331, https://1ref.us/1yf (accessed June 2, 2022).

67 Seyed Davoodi et al., "Health-Related Aspects of Milk Proteins," *Iranian Journal of Pharmaceutical Research* 13, no. 3 (Summer 2016): 573–591, https://1ref.us/1yg (accessed June 2, 2022).

Whey protein consists of globular proteins. Twenty percent Alpha-Lactalbumin (α-LA) and 50 percent beta-lactoglobulin (β-LG) are the predominant whey proteins and make up about 70–80 percent of the total whey proteins. Other types of whey proteins include immunoglobulins (Igs), serum albumin, lactoferrin (LF), lactoperoxidase (LP), and protease-peptones.

Casein is problematic to health because it is associated with the growth and development of cancer which may be due in part to the increased presence of circulating Insulin-like growth factor-1 (or IGF-1), a hormone that promotes cell growth and division in both normal and cancer cells with an increase in casein. Casein also has the distinction of being a major ingredient of some glues!

The ingestion of meat and milk products may provide the "complete" protein, but they are in amounts far greater than humans require. The problem then becomes one of excess protein. Therefore, the real problem is not a lack of protein but rather an excess of protein! People in the U.S. consume more than two to three times the amount of protein they need. Rather than falling prey to what I would coin the "hypoproteinaphobic" mentality, we really should be "hyperproteinaphobic," fearful of eating too much protein!

Those on a quest to get a large amount of protein each day are wasting food because the body does not use excess protein, it is stored. Instead, the ingestion of excess protein leads to a host of other problems, obesity being chief among them. Excess protein leads to an excessive amount of nitrogen when protein is broken down for digestion. The excess nitrogen can accumulate in the muscles and act as a kinotoxin (a fatigue toxin). The kidneys and liver are forced to work overtime to rid the body of the toxins and toxic levels of chemicals that result from excess protein ingestion.

Another consequence of excess protein consumption is the disease known as osteoporosis. With osteoporosis the bones lose calcium and therefore become more porous and softer. This condition of the bones leads to an increased susceptibility to fractures. When excess protein is consumed, the body requires additional calcium and gets it from the bones. Researchers at several universities have found that in the U.S., the meat-eating capital of the world, by the age of sixty-five, male meat-eaters have an average measurable bone loss of 7 percent, female meat-eaters have a measurable bone loss of 35 percent. Male vegetarians have a measurable bone loss of 3 percent, and female vegetarians have a measurable bone loss of 18 percent.

By knowing the amount of protein and calories in each food item, the percentage of calories in the form of protein for that particular food item can be calculated. This method of nutritional analysis is instrumental in determining the percentage of calories in the form of protein that is needed in the diet. For adults, the percentage of calories in the form of protein is well below 10 percent. In other words, if, according to the National Research Council, your daily diet should consist of sixty grams of protein and 3,000 calories (about 240 minutes (about 4 hours) of running), the percentage of protein in the form of calories that you require is only 8 percent. Virtually all plant items are composed of 10 to 49 percent protein. In other words, if you ate nothing but carrots in order to get your 3,000 calories (about 240 minutes of running), you would have 10 percent of the calories in the form of protein; this would be well more than the 8 percent calculated. Furthermore, if you ate nothing but spinach to get the same 3,000 calories, you would have 49 percent of your calories in the form of protein!!! Who says you need to eat dead animals in order to get "adequate" amounts of protein?????

By knowing the amount of protein and calories in each food item, the percentage of calories in the form of protein for that particular food item can be calculated.

Now, you are probably wondering if there is a difference in the quality of protein derived from animals and protein derived from plants. Interestingly enough, the debate over the quality of vegetable protein versus animal protein started more than seventy-five years ago, when researchers noticed that rats on a diet of certain vegetable proteins did not grow as fast as rats on an animal protein diet unless they were supplemented with certain amino acids.

At first glance, this seems to be quite an incredible discovery. It would appear that accelerated growth would be advantageous. Rapid growth beyond what is normal on a natural diet is not advantageous or something to be desired. "A diet giving the maximum rate of growth is not best for a long-life span. Rapid growth and short life go together" (Journal of American Medical Association, 171; 1959; p. 461). "...the general results of the Stanford, the Cornell, and the Columbia experiments consistently indicate that high protein intake increases the rate of growth but does not conduce to higher health or longer life." (Sherman, H.C., Science of Nutrition, 1943; p. 198).

In many growth studies, cow's milk is frequently used to give a high quality and quantity of protein that accelerates the growth of the subjects under study. Milk has been called "Nature's most perfect food." This is true only for species receiving milk from the same species, not from another species. When you compare the milk from a cow and that from a human, you will see that cow's milk is designed for calves and human milk for baby humans. Cow's milk has about 6 percent protein, while human milk during the first week of breastfeeding is 2 percent protein. During the second week, a mother's milk has 1.6 percent protein. The decrease in the percent of protein continues until the eighth week, when it is 1.2 percent protein. This demonstrates that cow's milk has three to five times the amount of protein as human milk. Humans grow much slower and live much longer than cows. The human growth period is about eighteen years with a life expectancy of seventy to ninety years. The growth period of a cow is two to three years, and its life expectancy is about sixteen years.

A newborn calf weighs about eighty-six pounds and will gain two and one-half pounds a day drinking its mother's milk. By the time it is weaned from its mother's milk, it will weigh about 600 pounds!!! By the time the calf is one year old, it will weigh about 700 pounds! As you can see, the milk from a cow is designed for rapid and explosive growth. Within a year, a cow 8is eight times its birth weight!

The average newborn human weighs seven and one-half pounds, and by the time it is one year of age, it will weigh twenty pounds, not quite tripling its birth weight. The average fully grown cow brain weighs between 450 to 500 grams or just under one pound. This means that in relation to its body, the brain of a cow is only about 0.1 percent. Conversely, the weight of a human brain at birth is 350 to 400 grams or about three-quarters of a pound. The brain of a fully developed person weighs 1,300 to 1,400 grams, or about 4 percent of the body weight. The difference in the relative size of the brain of the human is that it is forty times larger than the brain of a cow, even though a cow can easily weigh twenty times more than a human. This should make the case clear that cow's milk is designed for cows and not humans! Again, the composition of cow's milk is for rapid growth of the body and slow growth of the brain. The opposite is true of human breast milk; it is for a rapidly growing brain and slow body growth.

In addition to the multitudinous errors that may accompany this research on the growth of rats, the assumption is made that rats have the same protein requirements as humans! Needless to say, the protein requirements of rats differ considerably from humans! For instance, human babies can live off their mother's milk that has approximately 6 percent of its calories in the form of protein. Baby rats cannot live off human milk. Therefore, would we be correct in saying that human milk is not sufficient for the growth of human babies because it is not sufficient for the growth of baby rats??? NO!!! It is this faulty reasoning that has been the platform for the debate over the quality of protein for the past seventy-five-plus years. Protein is protein, and as such, I do not think that it is a question of the quality of the protein, but rather what it takes to get the protein. You can debate the quality of protein ad infinitum, but the critical issue with respect to the source of protein is what goes along with it. When you drink milk to get protein, you also get a lot of garbage as well. Drinking milk to get protein is like drinking sewage to get water. Consequently, the focus should shift from the isolated arena of amino acids and protein to the larger picture of the consequences of drinking the milk of cows and of other animals, such as goats.

There are many errors made in using cow's milk as a source of protein. For some reason, we think that animal protein is human protein. Once inside our body, the animal protein must be broken down into amino acids. The body then uses these amino acids as it sees fit. Furthermore, if you genuinely want protein from the animal, you must drink the milk from the cow raw. Pasteurizing milk destroys the amino acids that make up the protein!

There are many sources of protein besides milk. Weaned cows do not drink milk, yet they require a major source of protein. Where do they get their protein? Where do they get their "essential" amino acids? Consider elephants, oxen, mules, camels, water buffalo, and gorillas; they are some of the strongest animals around, yet they do not require milk once weaned. Where do they get their protein? They get their protein from plant sources! Incidentally, only 2–9 percent of the protein animals consume is returned in the form of meat. So not only are plant sources a more efficient source of protein, but they are also better. Why eat a dead cow to get expensive "sewage protein"?

Where can you get protein besides from dairy or animal flesh? You can get protein from beets, broccoli, cabbage, carrots, cauliflower, celery, collard greens, corn, cucumbers, eggplant, kale, lettuce, mushrooms, okra, onions, potatoes, pumpkins, radishes, spinach, squash, sweet potatoes, tomatoes, turnips, watercress, lima beans, pinto beans, chickpeas, lentils, peas, peanuts, soybeans, barley, bulgur, millet, oats, brown rice, wheat, almonds, cashews, pecans, sesame seeds, sunflower seeds, black walnuts, apples, avocados, bananas, blackberries, blueberries, cherries, grapes, lemons, oranges, peaches, pears, etc., etc. The point that I am trying to make is that every plant, seed, root, and fruit contains protein.

If you are one of those "essential" amino acid worriers, all fruits and vegetables contain most of the eight "essential" amino acids. However, potatoes, sweet potatoes, carrots, corn, bananas, cabbage, all nuts, cauliflower, sunflower seeds, eggplant, brussels sprouts, cucumbers, kale, peas, beans, sesame seeds, summer squash, and tomatoes contain all of the amino acids that your body needs. Soybeans are the best source of protein. They have all of the amino acids in amounts that the body needs.

Many people are under the misconception that protein is a major energy source. Generally, only in cases of severe starvation will the body utilize protein as its major source of energy. This is done only as a last resort since, by this time, the body's supply of carbohydrates and lipids (fats) have been used up. At this point, the body has no choice but to utilize the only remaining source of energy that it has—protein.

The ingestion of copious amounts of protein for the sake of acquiring a supply of energy actually has an adverse effect in supplying energy needs as well as a deleterious effect on your health. Protein is the most complex of all food elements and is the most difficult to break down. The body does not store protein. Excess protein is stored as fat. Proteins are broken down into amino acids and utilized as needed by the body. When the body has excess protein, the result is excess amino acids that result in nitrogenous waste products that the kidneys flush out with water, which can easily result in dehydration. The presence of nitrogenous waste products places an added strain on the liver and kidneys. The strain on the kidneys and liver is exacerbated by the added waste products in meat. This can be problematic in individuals with existing kidney issues or disease. Rather than gaining energy, as many have supposed, you actually end up wasting energy digesting excess protein. It would be like taking ten steps backward for every one step that you want to go forward. Now you know why lions spend 80 percent of their time asleep!

Chapter 7

MILK, IT DOES A CALF'S BODY GOOD, BUT NOT YOURS!

The dairy industry had a media campaign with the slogan "Milk, it does a body good!" What they did not tell you is that the only body milk that does good is that of a calf! When humans consume the milk of a cow, they do so to their own peril. It is hard to make it any plainer. Humans are not cows and should not be drinking milk from cows or from any other species, period! Many people do drink milk because they have been exposed to so much propaganda touting milk as a necessity for strong bones and teeth as well as growing up to be healthy that they have come to believe this.

One of the extremely basic problems with milk is that of excess. Milk has excess hormones, excess protein, excess calcium, excess saturated fat, excess pus cells, excess bacteria, and excess cholesterol. As you will soon see, milk does not do a human body good, but BAD!!!

Milk lays the foundation for disease in many ways. One way that is rather significant is that the ingestion of milk leads to chronic inflammation throughout the body. Inflammation is associated with heart disease, Alzheimer's, and arthritis. It is likely that the inflammation is due to the sugars that coat the cells of humans and those that coat the cells of animals, specifically those with spinal cords.

There is one particular sugar that coats the cells of humans that is closely related to a sugar that coats the cells of animals. The sugar is called sialic acid. The major function of sialic acids and glycans (also called polysaccharides) on different cell types is to help the immune system distinguish between what is a part of you and what is not a part of you. Different tissues have tens to hundreds of millions of glycan chains on the outside of each cell that are capped by sialic acids.[68] Sialic acids comprise a family of dozens of naturally occurring derivatives of the nine-carbon sugar neuraminic acid (5-amino-3,5-dideoxy-D-*glycero*-D-galactononulsonic acid.[69] One member of the sialic acid family is N-acetylated to form N-acetylneuraminic acid (Neu5Ac), which is one of the most widespread forms of sialic acid and almost the only form found in humans. The other member of the sialic acid family is based on N-glycolylneuraminic acid (Neu5Gc), which is common in many animal species but not humans.[70] More interesting is that humans lack the enzyme that allows for the formation of neu5Gc from Neu5Ac.

When humans consume animal products, cells take in the Neu5GC, it is taken into the lysosomes, and then makes its way to the nucleus, then to the Golgi apparatus, then onto the surface of the cell. It is here, on the surface of the cell, that the varying levels of circulating IgM, IgG, and IgA antibodies attack the Neuro5GC glycans, which then leads to inflammation with particular impact on the tissue of the lung, liver, and colon.

Heart Disease

The human heart is perhaps the most important organ of the body with respect to supplying the energy needs required to sustain life. When the heart stops beating, certain death is just moments away. The key role and function of the heart is that of a pump. The human heart weighs ten to eleven ounces and is about the size of a fist. In a single day, it beats 100,000 times, and with each beat, pumps about 80 ml or one-third of a cup of blood to send the equivalent of roughly 2,000 gallons of blood through the 60,000 miles of blood vessels in the body of a child, and nearly

---

68 Meghan Altman and Pascal Gagneux, "Absence of Neu5Gc and Presence of Anti-Neu-5Gc Antibodies in Humans-An Evolutionary Perspective," *Frontiers In Immunology* 10 (April 30, 2019), https://1ref.us/1yh (accessed June 2, 2022).

69 Melanie Koehler et al., "Initial Step of Virus Entry: Virion Binding to Cell-Surface Glycans," *Annual Review of Virology* 7 (September 2020): 143–165, https://1ref.us/1yi (accessed June 2, 2022).

70 b Wang and J Brand-Miller, "The Role and Potential of Sialic Acid In Human Nutrition," *European Journal of Clinical Nutrition* 57, no. 11 (November 2003): 1351–1369, https://1ref.us/1yj (accessed June 2, 2022).

100,000 miles in an adult, making certain that each cell of the body receives adequate nutrition and the removal of its waste products.[71]

As a result of the energy-demanding task the heart must perform, it accordingly requires its share of nutrients. Even though the heart is roughly 0.4 percent of the body weight, it receives approximately 4 percent of the blood output via the coronary arteries. The heart consumes 70 to 80 percent of the oxygen available within the blood circulating through the coronary vessels.[72] The heart is limited in its ability to take a greater percentage of oxygen from the blood flow; therefore, if the heart demands more oxygen, as in the case of exercise or stress, it must be met by an increase in the amount of blood flowing through the coronary arteries.

Cow's milk is loaded with cholesterol, animal protein, lactose, calcium, and saturated fat. There is a positive correlation between the consumption of milk and cholesterol levels and heart disease. The Framingham Heart Study has over the years provided epidemiological evidence that high serum cholesterol is a risk factor in coronary heart disease (CHD). In this study of 2,282 men and 2,845 women who lived in Framingham, Massachusetts, the serum cholesterol levels of nearly all of the participants ranged from 150 to 300 mg/dl. The investigators found that low levels of serum cholesterol were associated with low levels of CHD. Conversely, high serum cholesterol levels were associated with high rates of CHD.[73]

The Multiple Risk Factor Intervention Trial (MRFIT) was a randomized, primary prevention trial, in which several coronary risk factors were modified and were noted in 12,866 high-risk men from a cohort of more than 360,000 men (about half the population of Vermont). The data from the trial showed that the association between high serum cholesterol and increased CHD death begins with serum cholesterol levels as low as 180 mg/dl.[74]

The Nobel Prize in Physiology or Medicine in 1985 was awarded to doctors Michael Brown and Joseph Goldstein for their research on cell

71 "Blood Vessels," The Franklin Institute, https://1ref.us/1yk (accessed June 2, 2022).

72 "Physiology Tutorial—Coronary Circulation," Atlas of Human Cardiac Anatomy, University of Minnesota, https://1ref.us/1yl (accessed June 2, 2022).

73 WB Kannel, WP Castelli, and Gordon T, McNamara, "PM: Serum Cholesterol, Lipoproteins, and the Risk of Coronary Heart Disease," The Framingham Study, *Ann Intern Med* 74 (1971):1–12.

74 Multiple Risk Factor Intervention Trial Research Group, "Multiple Risk Factor Intervention Trial: Risk Factor Changes and Mortality Results," *JAMA* 248 (1982): 1465–1477, https://1ref.us/1ym (accessed June 2, 2022).

surface proteins they named low-density lipoprotein (LDL) receptors. They discovered that individuals with low or no LDL receptors were susceptible to atherosclerosis (plaque formation in the artery) and consequently early CHD. This is due to the necessity of LDL receptors to transport LDL particles, which are responsible for atherosclerosis, to the liver to be excreted. The decrease in LDL receptors appears to be signaled by a diet high in cholesterol and saturated fats.[75]

The Lipids Research Clinics Coronary Primary Prevention Trial (CPPT) provided evidence that showed that by reducing elevated levels of serum cholesterol, there would be a concomitant reduction risk of CHD. The trial consisted of more than 3,800 middle-aged men with high cholesterol in a double-blind study. It was determined that the men who took a full dose of medication that was responsible for the sequestration of bile acid had a 25 percent decrease in serum cholesterol and close to 34 percent fewer coronary events than the placebo group.[76]

There are attempts to negate these studies and show that cholesterol has no effect on lifespan. What should be noted, however, is that there is a difference in using lifespan as a measurement and using CHD as a measurement.

Serum cholesterol, especially VLDL (very-low-density lipoprotein) and LDL (low-density lipoprotein), have been implicated in the development of cardiovascular disease via its role in atherosclerosis. Cholesterol is not soluble in water and therefore is unable to circulate freely in the bloodstream. Cholesterol manages to get around by attaching itself to substances known as lipoproteins. Lipoproteins are small lipid-protein complexes. Once attached, it is the lipoproteins that then transport the cholesterol throughout the body.

There are several types of lipoproteins: high-density lipoprotein (HDL), low-density lipoprotein (LDL), and very-low-density lipoprotein (VLDL). They are named based on their relative fat-protein composition. As the percentage of fat increases in the lipoprotein, its density will be lower. Conversely, as the percentage of protein increases, its density increases.

---

75 MS Brown, PT Kovanen, JL Goldstein, "Regulation of Plasma Cholesterol by Lipoprotein Receptors," *Science* 212 (1981): 628–635, https://1ref.us/1yn (accessed June 2, 2022).
76 MH Frick et al., "Helsinki Heart Study: Primary-Prevention Trial with Gemfibrozil In Middle-Aged Men with Dyslipidemia," *The New England Journal of Medicine* 317, no. 20 (November 12, 1987): 1237–1245, https://1ref.us/1yo (accessed June 2, 2022).

VLDLs come from the liver, and their job is to transport substances called triglycerides to the "fat" (adipose) cells in the body. After they deliver the triglycerides, the VLDLs are then converted to LDLs. The LDLs are rich in cholesterol, and their primary job is to take cholesterol to various tissues in the body. HDL, also rich in cholesterol, transports cholesterol from various tissues in the body to the liver.

Generally, high LDL levels are of concern because of the cholesterol deposits that are made in the wall of the arteries. High HDL levels are of much less concern and even considered good because the cholesterol that they contain is from tissues and destined to the liver, where it will be broken down.

The amount of saturated fat consumed in the diet plays a key role in the amount of cholesterol in the blood. Saturated fats actually encourage the liver to produce more cholesterol while at the same time keeping it from leaving the body. Unsaturated fats, on the other hand, work to rid the body of cholesterol.

When humans ingest milk and dairy products, the saturated fats and cholesterol from these substances can cause, over a period of time, a condition known as atherosclerosis. In atherosclerosis, an abnormal mass of fat known as an atheroma attaches to the wall of a blood vessel. If this condition is found in any of the coronary arteries, the flow of blood to the heart muscle can be interrupted. If the blood flow of the coronary arteries is impeded to a serious degree, symptoms of myocardial ischemia will appear. The symptom most pronounced during myocardial ischemia is pain in the chest area known as angina pectoris. As atheromas grow, they can reach a size where they completely block a blood vessel, or they can break apart and travel through the blood vessel and become lodged in such a manner as to completely block the flow of blood through the vessel. Furthermore, the presence of atheromas on the wall of the blood vessel is conducive to the formation of blood clots. Once a blood clot is formed, it is easy for it to continue to grow in size until it completely blocks the passageway of the vessel. When the coronary arteries are blocked in this manner, the condition is referred to as a coronary thrombosis.

The process of developing coronary heart disease usually occurs over an extended period of time with a series of gradual, subtle, insidious events. Milk is instrumental in this process because it is high in calcium and lactose. Lactose promotes the intestinal absorption of calcium. This combination of high calcium and lactose leads to the calcification of the large arteries. As the blood vessels become narrowed due to the fatty substances that are deposited in the walls (atherosclerosis), the blood vessels may also become hardened (arteriosclerosis), thereby losing their elasticity, making them prone to leakage and rupture. The consumption of saturated fats and cholesterol from milk and dairy products over an extended period of time leads to, and exacerbates, atherosclerosis and arteriosclerosis. Milk is also rich in a substance called xanthine oxidase. Xanthine oxidase has been implicated in playing a role in artery disease by lessening the amount of phospholipids in the heart and arteries.

The future looks bleak with respect to decreasing the incidence of heart disease significantly because approximately 70 percent of children who consume the typical American diet have fatty deposits in their coronary arteries by the time they are twelve years old!

The Framingham Heart Study is the largest study of heart disease in America thus far. The data from that study has identified sulfur-based amino acids as the key to the etiology of heart disease. As a result, current research has discovered a link between protein and vitamin B-6 with atherosclerosis. Studies that show a high correlation between the cholesterol in the diet and the blood

> *Approximately 70 percent of children who consume the typical American diet have fatty deposits in their coronary arteries by the time they are twelve years old!*

and the degree of atherosclerotic lesions also show a strong correlation between the intake of animal protein and atherosclerosis.

Methionine is an amino acid that the body does not produce. Consequently, it must be acquired from the diet. When methionine is ingested, it is broken down into a substance known as homocysteine. Vitamin B-6 is then required to further break down homocysteine. If homocysteine is not broken down further, it is excreted in the urine. Individuals with a deficiency of vitamin B-6 or a high concentration of homocysteine develop severe atherosclerosis.

In addition to containing cholesterol, milk also contains a large amount of protein which contains the amino acid methionine, which breaks down to homocysteine. The diet free of milk is instrumental in reducing total serum cholesterol levels and LDL levels and consequently decreases the risk of coronary artery disease. Furthermore, the absence of copious amounts of animal protein further decreases the risk of atherosclerosis.

Myocardial infarction, more commonly known as heart attack, is the result of the heart muscle not getting enough oxygen and nutrients. Usually, a myocardial infarction is the result of a coronary thrombosis in one or more of the coronary arteries that resulted in coronary occlusion, impeding the flow of blood to the heart. Depending upon the severity of the coronary occlusion and the number of coronary arteries occluded, anything from minor heart muscle damage to death may result. Coronary heart disease may also be complicated by many factors such as age, high blood pressure, and obesity.

Coronary heart disease is a common occurrence; it is the number one killer of men and women in the United States. There are approximately 16.3 million Americans aged twenty and older who have CHD. The prevalence for men is 8.3 percent and for women is 6.1 percent. Non-Hispanic white men have the highest prevalence of CHD at 8.5 percent, followed by non-Hispanic black men at 7.9 percent and Mexican-American men at 6.3 percent. For women, non-Hispanic black women have the highest rate of CHD at 7.6 percent, followed by non-Hispanic white women at 5.8 percent and Mexican-American women at 5.6 percent.[77]

For those under sixty-five, sudden deaths account for more than half of all coronary deaths in that group. To make the situation even more grim, for every fatal episode of coronary heart disease, there are two non-fatal but disabling episodes. One study shows 48.5 percent of all coronary heart disease deaths were sudden, occurring out of a hospital and without medical assistance in most cases. Of those fatalities, over half of those people had never experienced an episode of clinical coronary heart disease.

Atherosclerosis and arteriosclerosis also play a significant role in the development of the condition known as congestive heart failure. Congestive heart failure is the inability of the heart to pump enough blood to meet the demands of the body. The narrowed and inelastic blood vessels cause the heart to work harder than it would normally while at the same time it is not receiving the necessary blood flow to maintain the workload required of it. This inefficient circulation of blood causes many organs to become congested with blood and tissue fluid. When this

---

77 VL Roger et al., "Heart Disease and Stroke Statistics—2011 Update: A Report from the American Heart Association," *Circulation* 123, no. 4 (December 15, 2010): e18–e209, https://1ref.us/1yp (accessed June 2, 2022).

happens, a variety of problems may arise, depending upon the extent to which a particular organ is affected.

The lining of the normal coronary arteries produces a substance known as endothelium-derived relaxation factor, EDRF. EDRF causes the coronary arteries to dilate, thereby increasing blood flow to the heart. Coronary arteries that are atherosclerotic are not able to produce EDRF in normal amounts. Consequently, these arteries become hypersensitive to stress and result in the arteries constricting rather than dilating. This leads to a decrease in blood flow, thereby increasing the risk of a heart attack and exacerbating congestive heart disease.

Cerebral Vascular Disease

What is commonly known as "strokes" are more properly referred to as cerebral vascular accidents, or more succinctly, CVAs. Having a stroke is not an accident. A better and more meaningful term than stroke or CVA is "brain attack," similar in significance to "heart attack."

Each year in the United States, there are 800,000 new strokes. There is one new stroke every fortyseconds. Strokes are the fifth leading cause of death and the first leading cause of disability. There are two main types of strokes. The more common type is an ischemic stroke, which is caused by interruption of blood flow to the area of the brain beyond the point of interruption. Ischemic strokes account for 85 percent of all acute strokes. The remaining 15 percent of acute strokes are hemorrhagic strokes. These are caused by the bursting of a blood vessel, i.e., acute hemorrhage.[78]

The damage done by a stroke is due to the result of the brain cells not receiving their much-needed supply of oxygen and nutrients. After their deprivation of oxygen and nutrients, these cells will die, and unlike other cells in the body, brain cells will not regenerate.

As stated earlier, in atherosclerosis, the passageway of the blood vessel becomes narrowed because of the atheromas attaching to and accumulating on the wall of the blood vessel. This action changes the normally smooth surface of the wall of the blood vessel to a rough one, thereby making the surface conducive for the formation of blood clots. Once blood clots form, they tend to continue to grow. As platelets become

---

78 P. Tadi and F. Lui, "Acute Stroke," NIH Stat Pearls, April 12, 2022, https://1ref.us/1yq (accessed June 2, 2022).

enmeshed in the fibronin threads, the platelets start to disintegrate. This results in the release of more thromboplastin, which, in turn, causes more clotting, which enmeshes more platelets, and so on, resulting in a vicious circle. These clots can continue to grow until they finally block the passageway of the blood vessel completely. Furthermore, these clots can break off and travel freely through the blood vessel until they become lodged on the wall and grow to form another large clot. This is particularly dangerous when it happens in the brain because of the many small blood vessels contained in it, the inability of modern medicine to reach these impaired vessels, and the inability of the brain cells to regenerate.

Atherosclerosis can also play a key role in cerebral vascular accidents when atheromas collect on the wall of blood vessels in the brain and continue to grow. If the growth of these atheromas continues uninterrupted, they will eventually block the flow of blood through the vessel completely or to a serious degree. In addition, the atheromas can break off and travel through the blood vessels of the brain freely, as in the case of blood clots, until they become lodged, thereby restricting the flow of blood, resulting in a cerebral vascular accident or stroke.

A study to explore the risk of strokes from dairy consumption was done on a group of 26,556 Finnish male smokers, none of whom had a history of strokes. They were followed for a period just under fourteen years. During that time, the researchers noted 2,702 cerebral infarctions, 383 intracerebral hemorrhages, and 196 subarachnoid hemorrhages within the group. The researchers concluded that there were associations between whole milk intake and stroke, which suggests that intake of certain dairy foods may be associated with the risk of stroke.[79]

Strokes result in the death of areas in the brain. These dead areas will not regenerate and will be replaced by scar tissue. Depending upon the amount and the area of the brain that was damaged, strokes may leave their victims completely or partially paralyzed. An individual suffering from a stroke may also experience a condition known as hemianopsia, the ability to see only half of their normal visual field.

---

79 Susanna Larsson et al., "Dairy Foods and Risk of Stroke," *Epidemiology* 20, no. 3 (May 2009): 355–360, https://1ref.us/1yr (accessed June 2, 2022).

New variant Creutzfeldt Jakob Disease (vCJD)

Creutzfeld-Jakob disease is a progressive, fatal degenerative spongiform disease of the brain. It is characterized by progressive dementia, massive incoordination, spastic dysarthria (imperfect articulation of speech due to disturbances of muscular control), and seizures.

This disease has gained considerable notoriety because of the BSE (bovine spongiform encephalopathy, also known as Mad Cow Disease) crisis in the U.K. as well as in the U.S. Approximately 4.4 million cattle were destroyed and incinerated during the Mad Cow disease crisis in Europe.[80] The ashes from these animals are stored because the organism responsible for BSE is still viable! One concern is that BSE appears to be transmissible to humans who consume infected beef, perhaps lamb and mutton as well. Recently, there have been several cases of a variant of CJD found in younger people, even teenagers, hence vCJD. The youngest known death due to vCJD was that of a fifteen-year-old girl in the U.K. CJD was thought to be a disease limited to those of middle age and beyond.

Given the lengthy incubation period of ten to forty years, many in the scientific community are bracing themselves for a possible epidemic of vCJD in the not-too-distant future. Since CJD and vCJD can only be confirmed by an autopsy, could it be that the alarming increase in the number of cases of what we loosely call Alzheimer's disease and dementia are actually misdiagnosed and undiagnosed cases of vCJD or CJD in various stages resulting from eating BSE infected meat and dairy???

BSE may be the preventable plague of the next millennium. There is so much to learn about BSE. Unfortunately, this book can only offer the tip of the tip of the proverbial iceberg of information on the topic. For considerably more information on the topic, the reader is strongly encouraged to read the books entitled *Deadly Feasts* authored by Richard Rhodes and published by Touchstone, and *Mad Cows and Milk Gate* by Virgil Hulse, published by Marble Mountain Publishing.

I've fallen down, and I can't get up! Osteoporosis

Osteoporosis, also known as "brittle bones," is fast becoming one of the leading degenerative diseases in the US. It affects nearly half of all

---

80 "'Mad Cow Disease': What Is BSE?" BBC News, October 18, 2018, https://1ref.us/1ys (accessed June 2, 2022).

women over the age of forty-five and nearly 90 percent of all women over seventy-five. Currently, there are about 54 million Americans who have osteoporosis and low bone mass, placing them at increased risk for osteoporosis. Studies suggest that approximately one in two women and up to one in four men age fifty and older will break a bone due to osteoporosis. Osteoporosis is responsible for two million broken bones and $19 billion (about $58 per person in the US) in related costs every year. By 2025, experts predict that osteoporosis will be responsible for approximately three million fractures, a 50 percent increase over current levels and $25.3 billion (about $78 per person in the US) in costs annually.[81]

There are two types of osteoporosis, type I and type II. Type I osteoporosis is characterized by a rapid loss of bone mass, usually of the trabecular, lattice of calcium-containing crystals, bone. It is in the trabecular where calcium is stored and subsequently withdrawn and placed in circulation when the blood levels of calcium are low. When the circulating levels of calcium are high, the excess calcium is placed back into the trabecular. Generally, the trabecular provides more than enough calcium for a lifetime; however, under certain conditions of long-term calcium depletion, the trabecular's supply of calcium diminishes to a crucial level resulting in weak, brittle bones. The bones are often so weak, especially in those over the age of sixty-five, that the vertebrae often disintegrate, causing pain due to the pinching of nerves. Teeth become loose and fall out due to the loss of calcium in the jawbone.

Type II osteoporosis is characterized by the withdrawal of calcium from cortical, dense bone that forms the exterior shell of a bone and the shaft of long bones, as well as the trabecular bone. The process of calcium withdrawal in type II is much slower in type II than in type I. Two of the key characteristics of type II osteoporosis are the compression of the spinal column due to the weakening of the vertebrae and fractures of the hip due to weakening of the shell and the interior of the bone. It is not unusual for a person to lose several inches in height due to the compression of the spinal cord.

One of the major causes of osteoporosis appears to be the excessive consumption of dietary protein. Countries with the highest rates of osteoporosis, such as the United States, England, and Sweden,

---

81 "What Is Osteoporosis and What Causes It?" Bone Health and Osteoporosis Foundation, https://1ref.us/1yt (accessed June 2, 2022).

interestingly, also consume the most milk. In contrast, China and Japan, where people eat low amounts of protein and dairy food, are among those that have the lowest rates of osteoporosis in the world. Worldwide, the highest rates of hip fractures are among populations that consume the most animal food (including dairy products), like people from the USA, Canada, Norway, Sweden, Australia, and New Zealand. The lowest rates are among people who eat little or no dairy foods like people from rural Asia and rural Africa. It should also be noted that human milk has only .9g protein per 100 ml; cow's milk has 3.3g of protein per 100 ml, nearly four times the amount of human milk.

A study regarding protein and osteoporosis examined the diets of 1,035 women, particularly focusing on the protein intake from animal and vegetable products. The study found that women with a high animal-to-vegetable protein ratio experienced an increased rate of femoral neck bone loss. A high animal-to-vegetable protein ratio was also associated with an increased risk of hip fracture. The author of the study stated, "Sulphur-containing amino acids in protein-containing foods are metabolized to sulfuric acid. Animal foods provide predominantly acid precursors. Acidosis stimulates osteoclastic activity and inhibits osteoblast activity." Moreover, the author of the study also noted, "Women with high animal-to-vegetable protein rations were heavier and had higher intake of total protein. These women had a significantly increased rate of bone loss than those who ate just vegetable protein. Women consuming higher rates of animal protein had higher rates of bone loss and hip fracture by a factor of four times."[82]

Calcium is, of course, in the spotlight when it comes to osteoporosis. The dairy industry is constantly pushing for the consumption of milk for strong bones. However, plants are also a source of calcium. Where do you think cows get theirs?

> *Women consuming higher rates of animal protein had higher rates of bone loss and hip fracture by a factor of four times.*

The answer to osteoporosis is not to be found in increasing your intake of calcium to excess by taking calcium supplements or by drinking

---

82 Study of Osteoporotic Fractures Research Group, "A High Ratio of Dietary Animal to Vegetable Protein Increases the Rate of Bone Loss and the Risk of Fracture in Post-menopausal Women," *The American Journal of Clinical Nutrition* 73, no. 1 (January 2001): 118–122, https://1ref.us/1yu (accessed June 2, 2022).

excessive amounts of milk since cow's milk has more than four times the calcium, 120mg per 100ml, than human milk has, 28mg per 100 ml. The percentage or bioavailability of calcium from milk is approximately 20 to 30 percent. Even when eating 1,400 mg of calcium daily, one can still lose up to 4 percent of his or her bone mass each year if they are consuming a high-protein diet! Research has demonstrated that excess protein causes a decrease in the amount of calcium in the body due to excretion of calcium in the urine.

A study in which calcium intake was 500 mg per day and protein intake varied from 47 to 95 to 142 g per day showed the relationship between calcium intake and high protein intake. When the protein intake was 47 g per day the mean calcium retention of the subjects was 31 mg. When the protein intake was 95 and 142 g, the mean calcium balance was -58 and -120 mg. Even by increasing the amount of fruits and vegetables by 50 percent there was no beneficial effect on calcium balance. The urinary calcium increased significantly with each increase in protein intake.[83]

Dietary protein increases production of acid in the blood, which is then often neutralized by calcium taken from the bones. Again, the ingestion of animal products with their large amounts of protein plays a crucial role in the development of osteoporosis. Conversely, diets low in protein tend to conserve calcium.

Calcium in bones tends to dissolve into the bloodstream then pass through the kidneys into the urine. Sodium (salt) in the foods you eat can greatly increase calcium loss through the kidneys. If you reduce your sodium intake to one to two grams per day, you will hold onto calcium better.

Many people may very well think that they are benefitting from consuming milk to build their bones, but given the above, the opposite is likely true. The low bioavailability of calcium in milk coupled with the high protein in milk leads to a negative calcium balance, not a positive one.

Cells that make up bone are called osteoblasts, and they are instrumental in the absorption of calcium. Osteoclasts, on the other hand, take calcium from the bones. Estrogen has an inverse relationship to bone

---

83 Chander Rekha Anand and Hellen M. Linkswiler, "Effect of Protein Intake on Calcium Balance of Young Men Given 500 mg Calcium Daily," *The Journal of Nutrition* 104, no. 6 (June 1974): 695–700, https://1ref.us/1yv (accessed June 2, 2022).

formation. Low levels of estrogen cause more calcium to be absorbed into the bones; this then leads to an increase in the production of osteoblasts and osteoclasts.[84][85][86][87][88] When the intake of calcium increases, the rate of calcium being removed is also increased. However, the majority of the osteoblasts die in the process of composing the new bone matrix.[89] The death of osteoblasts is prevented by estrogen.[90]

American women are in a group that consumes the largest amount of calcium in the world. What the dairy does not want you to realize is that American women also have one of the highest levels of osteoporosis in the world! When you examine the dietary habits and fractures in and around the world, the occurrence of osteoporosis revealing. Chinese people tend not to eat and drink dairy products, so they get all their calcium from vegetables. Though the Chinese consume only half the calcium of Americans, osteoporosis is not common in China. In South Africa, Bantu women who eat mostly plant protein and consume about 200-350mg of calcium a day have virtually no osteoporosis. This is of import because they have on average six children and breastfeed them. Conversely, African-Americans in the U.S. consume on average more than 1,000mg of calcium per day and are nine times more likely to experience hip fractures. The

84 RG Erben et al., "Androgen Deficiency Induces High Turnover Osteopenia in Aged Male Rats: A Sequential Histomorphometric Study," *Journal of Bone and Mineral Research* 15, no. 6 (June 2000): 1085–1098, https://1ref.us/1yw (accessed June 2, 2022).

85 P.Garnero et al., "Increased Bone Turnover in Late Postmenopausal Women Is a Major Determinant of Osteoporosis," *Journal of Bone and Mineral Research* 11, no. 3 (March 1996): 337–349, https://1ref.us/1yx (accessed June 2, 2022).

86 Y. Taguchi et al., "Interleukin-6-Type Cytokines Stimulate Mesenchymal Progenitor Differentiation Toward the Osteoblastic Lineage," *Proceedings of the Association of American Physicians* 110, no. 6 (Nov–Dec 1998): 559–574, https://1ref.us/1yy (accessed June 2, 2022).

87 RL Jilka et al., "Loss of Estrogen Upregulates Osteoblastogenesis In the Murine Bone Marrow," *The Journal of Clinical Investigation* 101, no. 9 (May 1, 1998): 1942–1950, https://1ref.us/1yz (accessed June 2, 2022).

88 KR Tau et al., "Estrogen Regulation of a Transforming Growth Factor-Beta Inducible Early Gene that Inhibits Deoxyribonucleic Acid Synthesis in Human Osteoblasts," *Endocrinology* 139, no. 3 (March 1998): 1346–1353, https://1ref.us/1z0 (accessed June 2, 2022).

89 RL Jilka et al., "Osteoblast Programmed Cell Death (Apoptosis): Modulation by Growth Factors and Cytokines," *Journal of Bone and Mineral Research* 13, no. 5 (May 1998): 793–802, https://1ref.us/1z1 (accessed June 2, 2022).

90 E Vegeto et al., "Estrogen and Progesterone Induction of Survival of Monoblastoid Cells Undergoing TNF-Alpha-Induced Apoptosis," *FASEB Journal* 13, no. 8 (May 1999): 793–803, https://1ref.us/1z2 (accessed June 2, 2022).

association between the consumption of animal protein and fracture rates is undeniable.

The Chinese population serves as an interesting example of diet and fracture risk. Americans consume more cow's milk than most countries in the world, and US women over the age of fifty have the distinction of having one of the highest rates of osteoporosis in the world.[91] The traditional diet of the Chinese has been associated with one of the lowest hip fracture rates in the world.[92] Hip fracture rates is one indicator of bone strength and osteoporosis. Studying and gathering data on Chinese women has brought remarkable results. One such body of information, the Bejing Osteoporosis project, shows that women in Beijing, China had a hip fracture rate that was less than 20% of that seen in White women in the United States. Additionally, the hip fracture rate in American men was more than twice that of Chinese men.[93] The difference in fracture rates, it seems, can largely be attributed to diet, in particular, the consumption of animal protein. For instance, cross-cultural studies show a positive relationship between the consumption of animal protein and the risk of hip fracture.[94]

The western diet is creeping into Asia as the food corporations and meat and dairy industry seek to enter burgeoning markets. As these entities encroach more and more into the Chinese diet, there will be no health benefit, only detriment. Already, the areas of mainland China where the traditional Chinese diet has given way to the western diet are showing increased hip fracture rates. Elderly women whose diets contain a high ratio of animal to vegetable protein have more rapid bone loss and greater risk for hip fracture compared with those with a low ratio of animal to vegetable protein.[95]

---

91 LA Frassetto, KM Todd, RC Morris Jr, A. Sebastian, "Worldwide Incidence of Hip Fracture in Elderly Women: Relation to Consumption of Animal and Vegetable Foods," *The Journals of Gerontology. Series A, Biological Sciences and Medical Sciences* 55, no. 10 (October 2000): M585–M592, https://1ref.us/1z3 (accessed June 2, 2022).
92 X Ling et al., "Very Low Rates of Hip Fracture in Beijing, People's Republic of China: The Beijing Osteoporosis Project," *Journal of American Epidemiology* 144, no. 9 (November 1996): 901–907, https://1ref.us/1z4 (accessed June 2, 2022).
93 Ling, "Ver Low Rates of Hip Fracture," 901–907.
94 BJ Abelow, TR Holford, KL Insogna, "Cross-Cultural Association Between Dietary Animal Protein and Hip Fracture: A Hypothesis," *Calcified Tissue International* 50, no. 1 (January 1992): 14–18, https://1ref.us/1z5 (accessed June 2, 2022).
95 DE Sellmeyer et al., "A High Ratio of Dietary Animal to Vegetable Protein Increases the Rate of Bone Loss and the Risk of Fracture in Postmenopausal Women," *The Ameri-*

Research is out now that shows that getting more than about 600 milligrams of calcium per day, surprisingly, does nothing to make bones stronger.[96] What is quite surprising is that research also shows that the consumption of dairy products are basically of no benefit to the bones of children.[97] One study showed that when researchers tracked the diets, exercise, and stress fracture rates of young girls for a period of seven years, they concluded that dairy products and calcium did not prevent stress fractures in these adolescent girls.[98]

Bones require more than just calcium for growth and repair. One such necessary factor for bones is vitamins, vitamins D and K specifically. Much has been discovered about leafy green vegetables like kale and broccoli. One of the benefits that these vegetables have is that they contain large amounts of calcium in addition to vitamins D and K. Vitamin D is instrumental in the absorption of calcium.[99] One of the selling points of milk is that it contains vitamin D. The reason why milk contains vitamin D is because it was added to the milk. Milk does not contain vitamin D naturally. Vitamin D is made by humans in our skin when sunlight hits it. On average it only takes a few minutes of sun exposure daily to acquire the proper amount of vitamin D. Consuming soy milk and various plant-based milks, and fortified orange juice will give you closely the same amount of calcium per serving as milk or other dairy products. Perhaps the easiest way to get the bones in shape is to exercise, and is one of the most effective ways to increase bone density and decrease the risk of osteoporosis.[100]

can Journal of Clinical Nutrition 73, no. 1 (January. 2001): 118–122, https://1ref.us/1z6 (accessed June 2, 2022).

96 D Feskanich, W Willett, G Colditz, "Calcium, Vitamin D, Milk Consumption, and Hip Fractures: A Prospective Study Among Postmenopausal Women," *The American Journal of Clinical Nutrition* 77, no. 2 (February 2003): 504–511, https://1ref.us/1z7 (accessed June 2, 2022).

97 A Lanou, S Berkow, N Barnard, "Calcium, Dairy Products, and Bone Health in Children and Young Adults: A Reevaluation of the Evidence," *Pediatrics* 115, no. 3 (March 2005): 736–743, https://1ref.us/1z8 (accessed June 2, 2022).

98 K Sonneville et al., "Vitamin D, Calcium, and Dairy Intakes and Stress Fractures Among Female Adolescents," *Archives of Pediatric and Adolescent Medicine* 166, no. 7 (July 2012): 595–600, https://1ref.us/1z9 (accessed June 2, 2022).

99 MF Holick and M Garabedian, "Vitamin D: Photobiology, Metabolism, Mechanism of Action, and Clinical Applications," in *Primer on the Metabolic Bone Diseases and Disorders of Mineral Metabolism,* 6th edition, edited by MJ Favus (Washington, D.C.: American Society for Bone and Mineral Research), 129–137.5.

100 T Lloyd et al., "Modifiable Determinants of Bone Status In Young Women," *Bone* 30, no. 2 (February 2002): 416–421, https://1ref.us/1za (accessed June 2, 2022).

Non-Alcoholic Fatty Liver Disease

Diets high in animal protein increase the risk for fatty liver disease among people who are overweight, according to new research published in *Gut*. Researchers compared intake of fiber, protein, and other macronutrients with liver disease incidence rates via ultrasounds in 3,882 participants from the Rotterdam Study. Results showed a 36 percent higher risk for fatty liver disease for those who consumed the most animal protein compared with those who consumed the least. The results showed no negative associations between carbohydrate consumption and liver disease. Suspected mechanisms behind the increased risk include nitrates, nitrites, and heme iron due to their influence on insulin resistance, endothelial function, and oxidative stress. The authors suggest preventive dietary recommendations shift focus toward protein in place of fat and carbohydrates.[101]

Diabetes Mellitus

Diabetes is a serious disease and is increasing in prevalence at an alarming rate. It is the leading cause of non-trauma amputation. In 1990, there were only 6.2 million people (about twice the population of Nevada) who were diagnosed with diabetes. By 2000, that number had almost doubled by jumping up to just over 12 million people (about twice the population of Arizona).[102] In 2018, the number climbed to 34.2 million, or 10.5 percent of the population. Nearly 1.6 million Americans have type 1 diabetes, including about 187,000 children and adolescents. Of the 34.2 million adults with diabetes, 26.8 million were diagnosed, and 7.3 million were undiagnosed. The percentage of Americans who are sixty-five and older with diabetes is 26.8 percent, or 14.3 million seniors (diagnosed and undiagnosed). Each year, 1.5 million Americans are diagnosed with diabetes. In 2015, 88 million Americans age eighteen and older had prediabetes. About 210,000 Americans under age twenty are estimated to have diagnosed diabetes, approximately 0.25 percent of that population.

101 Louise Alferink et al., "Association of Dietary Macronutrient Composition and Non-Alcoholic Fatty Liver Disease In an Ageing Population: The Rotterdam Study," *Gut* 68, no. 6 (June 2019): 1088–1098, https://1ref.us/1zb (accessed June 2, 2022).
102 "Number of US Americans with Diagnosed Diabetes from 1980 to 2019 (In Millions)," Statista, https://1ref.us/1zc (accessed June 2, 2022).

In 2014–2015, the annual incidence of diagnosed diabetes in youth was estimated at 18,200 with type 1 diabetes and 5,800 with type 2 diabetes.[103]

Diabetes is an equal opportunity disease and does not discriminate along racial lines, though some groups are affected more than others. For instance, diabetes is found in 7.4 percent of non-Hispanic whites, 9.5 percent of Asian Americans, 11.8 percent of Hispanics, 12.1 percent of non-Hispanic blacks,14.5 percent of American Indians/Alaskan Natives.[104] The most common characteristic of diabetics is obesity. Approximately 85 percent of the people with diabetes are obese.[105] Type II diabetes also has in common with type I diabetes, polyuria (frequent urination), polydipsia (excessive thirst), and polyphagia (excessive eating). In addition, individuals will suffer with fatigue and tend to be irritable.

Diabetes was the seventh leading cause of death in the United States in 2017 based on the 83,564 death certificates in which diabetes was listed as the underlying cause of death. In 2017, diabetes was mentioned as a cause of death in a total of 270,702 certificates. These numbers appear to be high, but they may actually be low compared to the true number of cases. Diabetes may be underreported as a cause of death. Studies have found that only about 35 percent to 40 percent of people with diabetes who died had diabetes listed anywhere on the death certificate, and about 10 percent to 15 percent had it listed as the underlying cause of death.[106]

The acute complications of diabetes are hypoglycemia (low blood sugar), DKA (diabetic ketoacidosis), and HHNC (hyperglycemic hyperosmolar non-ketonic coma). Hypoglycemia can occur at any time. It is simply a decrease in the level of sugar in the blood. The classic signs are an increased heart rate, tremors, shaking, nervousness, sweating, headache, confusion, and slurred speech. In severe cases it can lead to seizures, a decreased level of consciousness, irreversible brain damage, and ultimately death.

DKA results from hyperglycemia leading to polyuria, which leads to polydipsia, which leads to dehydration. At this point, the body begins to break down fat. The breakdown of fat has as one of its by-products ketones.

---

103 "Statistics About Diabetes," American Diabetes Association, https://1ref.us/1zd (accessed June 2, 2022).
104 "Statistics About Diabetes."
105 Alvin Powell, "Obesity? Diabetes? We've Been Set Up," *The Harvard Gazette,* March 7, 2012, https://1ref.us/1ze (accessed June 2, 2022).
106 "Statistics About Diabetes."

The amounts of ketones in the body increases as the fat is broken down. Increased levels of ketones cause acidosis. This condition is characterized by anorexia (decreased appetite), nausea, vomiting, and arrhythmias and is found in type I diabetes.

HHNC begins with hyperglycemia and ends in a non-ketonic coma. This is found in type II diabetes. The insulin that type II individuals possess is enough to prevent them from having ketosis. Hence, they will go into a non-ketonic coma if they are not treated in time. The symptoms of HHNC are profound dehydration, increased heart rate, decreased blood pressure, and lethargy. It is not unusual for people with HHNC to have blood sugars in excess of 2000!

There are long-term complications of diabetes. They are macrovascular and microvascular changes and infections. The macrovascular changes progress at a faster rate and at an earlier age in diabetics than non-diabetics. They are more common in type II diabetes. The major macrovascular changes are coronary artery disease, which accounts for over half of all deaths of diabetics, cerebral vascular accidents (CVA or stroke), and peripheral vascular disease (PVD).

The microvascular changes are retinopathy and nephropathy, both of which are more common in type I diabetes. Retinopathy results from blood vessels leaking blood and fluids in the retina of the eye. Scar tissue is formed that causes blurred vision and ultimately blindness. Nephropathy is damage to the kidney. Ultimately, this can lead to renal failure that would then require dialysis.

The decreased ability of the body to metabolize protein, fat, and carbohydrate as a result of decreased insulin production and/or resistance of target tissues to insulin characterize it. In other words, the part of the body that produces the insulin, the pancreas, is not working properly, and for whatever reason, the tissues (groups of specific cells) do not allow the insulin in.

The pancreas is a small organ that is about six inches long and two inches wide and weighs about three ounces. It is a unique organ in that it has an exocrine and endocrine function, making it act as though it is two separate organs. Its exocrine function is to produce digestive juices and enzymes that digest fats, proteins, and carbohydrates that will be absorbed through the intestine. Its endocrine function is to make hormones, one of which is insulin, which regulate the use and storage of glucose and fats, which are the main energy sources of the body.

Diabetes can be seen as the result of a pre-receptor defect, which means that the pancreas is not secreting any insulin due to destruction of the beta cells; as a receptor defect, in which case there is a decrease in the number of receptors on the cells and/or a decreased sensitivity to insulin; and finally, a post-receptor defect, in which case there is an enzymatic problem within the cell.

The major role of insulin, which is an anabolic hormone, is that of stimulating the liver to store the simple sugar glucose. Every cell in your body needs glucose in order to survive. The cell, as its primary source of energy, uses glucose. Insulin is also instrumental in enhancing the storage of fat from the diet into adipose tissue or "fat" cells and increasing the use of amino acids, which, in turn, decreases the breakdown of stored glucose, fat, and protein.

There are two major types of diabetes mellitus. Type I, which is also known as Juvenile Onset Diabetes and Insulin Dependent Diabetes Mellitus (IDDM). This group makes up 5 to 10 percent of all individuals with diabetes mellitus. Type II, which is also known as Adult-Onset Diabetes and Non-Insulin Dependent Diabetes Mellitus. This group makes up 90 to 95 percent of all individuals with diabetes mellitus.

Type I Diabetes Mellitus is characterized by a substantial decrease in the production of insulin. This decrease in the production of insulin is due to the immune system destroying B cells. It has an abrupt onset. Symptoms appear when approximately 70–90 percent of the insulin-producing cells are destroyed. This decreased amount of insulin leads to a condition known as hyperglycemia. Which is just a term meaning a high amount of glucose in the blood. When the blood sugar level gets in the range of 180, the kidneys begin to secrete glucose in the urine. At which point a whole chain of events begins to take place. The cells begin to secrete water that goes to the kidneys, which then dumps it out in the form of urine. This leads to a condition known as polyuria, which simply means a whole lot of urine. As you begin to urinate large amounts of urine, you will become dehydrated. Due to being dehydrated, you will begin to drink a lot of fluids that is a condition known as polydipsia. In the meantime, the cells are literally starving from not having any glucose. The starving cells plus the excess glucose in the blood makes you hungry, thereby causing you to eat more. That is known as polyphagia. Since the body is starved for energy, it begins to break down fat for energy. This process leads to the production of by-products called ketones. The increase of ketones in the blood leads to a condition known as metabolic acidosis. This, in turn, causes chemical changes in the brain, causing coma and ultimately death.

For years, it has been postulated that cow's milk is a possible cause of the autoimmune response that destroys the cells on the pancreas responsible for the production of insulin and thereby causing diabetes. Additionally, bovine serum albumin (BSA) is the protein in milk that is responsible. This was confirmed in a study that showed that patients with insulin-dependent diabetes mellitus are immune from the albumin found in cow's milk, and they have antibodies to an albumin peptide that can react with the beta cell-specific surface protein, which could ultimately lead to its destruction.[107]

Some studies have shown that abbreviated breastfeeding and the early introduction of milk in the first few years of a child's life increases the risk of diabetes one and a half times.[108] It is interesting to note that when a nursing mother drinks cow's milk, the proteins from the milk will be in her milk.[109]

One study showed that lymphocytes from a large proportion of patients with recent-onset IDDM increase rapidly in response to β casein, a finding that reinforces the concept that this protein is involved in causing the diabetes as seen by the recent report of autoantibodies to β casein in these patients.[110] "A proliferative response to β casein in patients with IDDM diagnosed in childhood and as young adults suggests that this response has pathogenic relevance regardless of the age of onset of the disease." This data and the observation that a high percentage of IDDM patients have antibodies to β casein indicate β casein as a good candidate milk protein related to IDDM.[111] In addition to β casein, intensified cellular

107 J Karjalainen et al., "A Bovine Albumin Peptide as a Possible Trigger of Insulin-Dependent Diabetes Mellitus," *The New England Journal of Medicine* 327, no. 5 (July 1992): 302–307, https://1ref.us/1zf (accessed June 2, 2022).

108 HC Gerstein, "Cow's Milk Exposure and Type I Diabetes Mellitus. A Critical Overview of the Clinical Literature," *Diabetes Care* 17, no. 1 (January 1994): 13–9, https://1ref.us/1zg (accessed June 2, 2022).

109 *Lancet* 348, no. 9032 (October 5, 1996): 905, https://1ref.us/1zh (accessed June 2, 2022).

110 HE Wasmuth, F Becker, S Seebaum, RB Elliot, K Fenderlin, "Association of Antibodies to β Casein with Type I Diabetes. Autoimmunity," 21 (1995): A328.

111 MG Cavallo, D Fava, L Monetini, F Barone, P Pozzilli, "Cell-Mediated Immune Response to Beta Casein In Recent-Onset Insulin-Dependent Diabetes: Implications for Disease Pathogenesis," *The Lancet* 348, no. 9032 (October 1996): 926–928, https://1ref.us/1zi (accessed June 2, 2022).

and humoral immune responses have been noted with other ingredients of cow's milk such as 3 lactoglobulin and bovine serum albumin.[112,113,114,115] Therefore, a role for β casein in the pathophysiology of IDDM may be easily seen.

In a study conducted by Dr. Johanna Paronen from University of Helsinki, Finland, after taking into account the differences in the timing of the introduction of supplemental milk between the randomization groups, the researchers found that at the age of three months, both cellular and humoral responses to bovine insulin were higher in infants exposed to cow's milk than in infants fully breastfed. IgG antibodies to bovine insulin were also higher in infants who received cow's milk than in infants who received the formula at three months of age.[116]

In addition, these responses were also higher for those infants receiving cow's milk than for fourteen infants whose mothers decided to continue exclusively breastfeeding their babies past eight months, never adding cow's milk or formula to their baby's diet. The results show that at three months of age, infants who had been fed cow's milk had a significantly higher immune response to bovine insulin than did infants who received the other formula or were breastfed, the authors reported.[117]

> *At three months of age, infants who had been fed cow's milk had a significantly higher immune response to bovine insulin than did infants who received the other formula or were breastfed*

---

112 MG Cavallo et al., "Cell-mediated Immune Response to β Casein In Recent-Onset Insulin-Dependent Diabetes: Implications for Disease Pathogenesis," *The Lancet* 348, no. 9032 (October 1996): 926–928, https://1ref.us/1zj (accessed June 2, 2022).

113 G Dahlquist, E Savilahti, M Landin-Olsson, "An Increased Level of Antibodies to β-Ltoglobulin Is a Risk Determinant for Early-Onset Type 1 (Insulin-Dependent) Diabetes Mellitus Independent of Islet Cell Antibodies and Early Introduction of Cow's Milk," *Diabetologia* 35 (October 1992): 980–984, https://1ref.us/1zk (accessed June 2, 2022).

114 J Karjalainen et al., "A Bovine Albumin Peptide as a Possible Trigger of Insulin-Dependent Diabetes Mellitus," *The New England Journal of Medicine* 327, no. 5 (July 1992): 302–307, https://1ref.us/1zf (accessed June 2, 2022).

115 I Miyazaki et al., "T Cell Activation and Anergy to Islet Cell Antigen In Type I Diabetes," *Journal of Immunology* 154, no. 3 (February 1995): 1461–1469, https://1ref.us/1zl (accessed June 2, 2022).

116 S Gottlieb, "Early Exposure to Cows' Milk Raises Risk of Diabetes In High Risk Children," *BMJ* 321, no. 7268 (October 2000): 1040D, https://1ref.us/1zm (accessed June 2, 2022).

117 Gottlieb, "Early Exposure to Cows' Milk."

Strengthening the connection between milk and diabetes is the strong correlation between total cow's milk consumption and type 1 diabetes found all over the world. For example, a country with a high milk-consuming population, such as the United States, has thirty-six times more type 1 diabetes than does Japan, a country with a low milk-consuming population. This relationship has also been found within a country. Italy, for example, has parts that consume large amounts of milk with higher rates of diabetes than those regions which consume lower amounts of dairy.

Antibodies that the body made specifically to attack and destroy the cow's milk protein also find and attach themselves to the beta cells, thereby activating T-cells, which then attack and destroy these insulin-producing cells and the foreign cow's milk proteins. As the number of beta cells destroyed increases, the ability of the pancreas to produce enough insulin to meet the body's needs decreases. Finally, when the beta cells are completely destroyed, the body can no longer produce insulin, and daily injections of insulin are then required to meet the needs of the body.

It may take years before the beta cells are completely destroyed. Once they are destroyed, they will not be able to be regenerated. Symptoms of diabetes generally appear suddenly and abruptly. Within a very short period of time, the person begins to have excessive thirst and urinates frequently. In addition, they become extremely tired. It is not unusual for a person to lapse into a coma or die at this time.

Type II diabetes has a slow onset. It is characterized by a decrease in the number of receptors on the cell for insulin and/or a marked insensitivity of the cell to insulin. Both of which lead to a decrease of insulin in the cell. Some insulin is still available and gets into the cell; it's just that it is not enough.

In industrialized countries where bottle-feeding is the norm, cow's milk proteins are typically the first foreign proteins to enter the gastrointestinal tract of infants since most infant formulas are cow's milk-based. The evidence is so compelling that in June of 1992, the American Academy of Pediatrics Committee on Nutrition recommended that cow's milk was not suitable as an alternative to breast milk for the first year of life.

The March 2005 issue of the European Journal of Clinical Nutrition contains a study by Hoppe, et al., which demonstrated that high intake of dairy products increased insulin resistance in eight-year-old boys. Eight-year-old boys were divided into three groups. Group one, the control group, did not consume meat or milk for one week. Members of group two consumed 53 grams of meat protein for one week. The members of group three were given 53 grams of milk protein for one week. During this week period, daily measurements of blood levels of insulin, glucose, and amino acids were taken. Then insulin resistance was calculated for each child. Insulin resistance is a condition that causes the body not to respond to the action of insulin hormone, although enough insulin is produced. This occurs often in people with type 2 diabetes. At the end of the study, the children in group three, the group that was given 53 grams of milk protein per day, insulin resistance doubled when compared to the control group, the group that did not consume milk or meat.

Researchers at the National Public Health Institute in Helsinki, Finland, did a study on diabetes. They studied 4,304 people who had not been previously diagnosed with diabetes during the study's baseline years of 1967–1972 of this twenty-three-year study. Subsequently, 383 of the participants were diagnosed with diabetes. They were divided into two groups, Group A and Group B. Group A had a high consumption of fruits and vegetables. Group B had a high consumption of milk, cheese, butter, and potatoes. Not surprisingly, the researchers concluded that those in Group A, the high consumers of fruits and vegetables, were associated with reduced risks of diabetes. Conversely, those in Group B, the high consumers of milk, cheese, butter, and potatoes, were associated with the higher risk of diabetes. The researchers concluded that "In light of these results, it appears that the risk of developing type 2 diabetes can be reduced by changing dietary patterns."[118]

Finland has the highest rate of diabetes in the world and the highest rate of milk and cheese consumption in the world. The average daily milk protein in Finland is 30 grams, compared to nineteen in the United States and five in Japan. Finland has the distinction of having almost double the rate of diabetes of the United States. More chilling is the fact that for every one case of diabetes in Japan, there are twenty-eight in Finland!!!

Cow's Milk Allergy

The intestine has openings that allow milk proteins to pass through and go directly into the bloodstream avoiding digestion. This is a normal

---

118 Jukka Montonen, *Plant Foods in the Prevention of Type 2 Diabetes Mellitus with Emphasis on Dietary Fiber and Antioxidant Vitamins* (Helsinki: Publications of the National Public Health Institute, 2005).

mechanism that allows immune globulin proteins from a mother's milk to get into a baby's system. However, the milk protein from a cow is different than that of human milk. The cow protein is seen as "foreign" by the human system since it is from a different animal species and, upon detection, stimulates the immune system to respond to their presence.

The immune system begins to make antibodies to the "foreign" proteins. The antibodies are used to destroy the invading foreign proteins. The foreign milk protein escaping the intestine can attach to cells in the body. When the "foreign" protein attaches to the cells, the antibodies end up destroying the cells to which the foreign proteins have attached and destroys them as well as the foreign protein.

The most common food allergy in young children is cow's milk allergy. Its closest rival is the common chicken egg. Most infants that are bottle-fed with cow's milk develop allergic symptoms indicative of rejection to cow's milk proteins within the first few weeks of birth. Studies have shown that such babies at the age of three months were secreting low levels of serum antibodies to cow proteins. The majority will have eczema, rashes, or other skin manifestations, gastrointestinal symptoms, retarded growth, and respiratory symptoms. In some cases, children may have a serious allergic reaction called anaphylaxis. This reaction will generally occur within minutes of consuming something the child is allergic to. Anaphylaxis can result in swelling of the face, mouth, and tongue that leads to the child having difficulty breathing. Hives, itch rash, and severe vomiting may also occur. Studies also show that infants who are fed a casein (cow milk protein) rich evaporated milk develop a disorder known as transient tyrosinemia. Tyrosinemia is a failure to properly metabolize the amino acid tyrosine, which results in learning disabilities.

Cow's milk protein allergy can develop in both breastfed and formula-fed children. However, breastfed children are usually less likely to develop food allergies of any sort. Occasionally, though, breastfed children develop cow's milk allergy when they react to the slight amount of cow's milk protein that is passed along from their mother's diet into her breast milk. In other cases, certain babies can become sensitized to the cow's milk protein in their mother's breast milk but don't actually have an allergic reaction until they are later introduced to cow's milk themselves. Fortunately, most babies outgrow milk allergies by the second or third year of their life. Currently, there is not an effective treatment on the market that can cure milk allergies. Even if such a cure did exist, would it not make a lot more sense to avoid the problem in the first place by simply eliminating dairy from the diet?

In this era of factory food, it is hard to have a diet that is completely free of milk protein because, thanks to the gallant efforts of the dairy industry to find a market for its junk, milk proteins are found, of course, in cottage cheese, sour cream, cheese, whey, yogurt, and milk. However, milk solids and sodium caseinate are milk proteins that are added to food.

Constipation

What are some of the factors that cause constipation? Generally, for years we were led to believe that constipation is chiefly the result of eating foods with little or no fiber. However, constipation also results from an inflamed colon.

A study that was published in the New England Journal of Medicine of sixty-five children who were severely constipated demonstrated the role that milk consumption played in constipation. The children in the study had a bowel movement once every three to fifteen days! When these children had cow's milk removed from their diet, forty-four of the sixty-five, 68 percent, were relieved of constipation. When their bowels were biopsied, inflammation was observed. The children were milk-free for eight to twelve months. When cow's milk was again introduced and made a part of their diet, all of the children developed constipation within five to ten days![119]

Anemia

Drinking cow's milk results in anemia because it causes bleeding in the intestines and thereby reduces the body's store of iron. It starts in infancy. Frank Oski, MD., former pediatrics director at Johns Hopkins University School of Medicine, estimated in his book *Don't Drink Your Milk!* that half of all iron deficiency in U.S. infants results from cow's milk-induced intestinal bleeding! More than 15 percent of American children under two years of age suffer from iron-deficiency anemia. American infants drink so

---

119 Giuseppe Iacono et al., "Íntolerance of Cow's Milk and Chronic Constipation In Children," *The New England Journal of Medicine* 339 (October 1998): 1100–1104, https://1ref. us/1zn (accessed June 2, 2022).

much milk, a substance that contains very little iron, that gastrointestinal bleeding is induced, which causes iron loss.

Acne

The Journal of the American Academy of Dermatology contained a study in February 2005 associated dairy products with acne. Harvard's School of Public Health did the study that investigated data from more than 47,000 women (about twice the seating capacity of Madison Square Garden). The results showed that those who drank three or more cups of milk a day were 22 percent more likely to experience severe acne compared with those who drank less than one serving a week. Other milk products such as cottage cheese and cream cheese were also associated with acne. There was even a stronger link between acne and milk consumption with skim milk. It was concluded that the hormones and other bioactive molecules were responsible for the episodes of acne.[120]

Gallstones

The gallbladder acts as a warehouse for bile. Bile is a substance manufactured in the liver and is secreted to the gallbladder for storage. The gallbladder then secretes the bile during the digestion of fats. There are several types of gallstones. By far the most common are those that are composed of cholesterol, which accounts for 80 percent of all gallstones. This indicates that cholesterol plays a key role in the formation of gallstones.

In order to grow, these cholesterol gallstones require bile with a high concentration of cholesterol. This type of bile allows small crystals to form. These small crystals attach to each other until a small stone finally develops. These stones can grow large enough to block the passageway between the gallbladder and the passageway from the liver to the small intestine. These stones may, in addition to blocking the passageways, damage the wall of the passageway and the wall of the gallbladder itself.

If the gallstones block the passageway between the gallbladder and the passageway from the liver to the small intestine, the affected person may

120 Clement Adebamowo et al., "High School Dietary Dairy Intake and Teenage Acne," *Journal of the American Academy of Dermatology* 52, no. 2 (February 2005): 207–214, https://1ref.us/1zo (accessed June 2, 2022).

experience a great amount of pain. The pain is the result of the muscles of the gallbladder contracting as they work to secrete bile, having the passageway blocked. This may lead to inflammation of the gallbladder, a condition known as cholecystitis. If the passageway from the liver to the small intestine is blocked by gallstones, jaundice and other problems may result due to the inability of the bile to leave the liver.

Kidney and Related Diseases

The excessive work our kidneys must perform when we eat meat is the result of two different sources. The first source is from the waste products of the animal you've eaten. Your kidneys are biological filters that filter your blood. When you eat animal flesh, you take into your system the waste products of that animal. Consequently, your kidneys not only have to take care of the waste that occurs naturally in your body, but they must also have the additional task of having to deal with the added waste products of the animal you ate. The second cause of overworked kidneys involves the high concentration and large amounts of animal protein in meat. When our bodies digest the protein from animal flesh, it results in the production of nitrogenous chemicals and urea.

When the kidneys are not functioning properly, chemicals such as urea, uric acid, creatine, and other nitrogenous chemicals build up in the bloodstream, a situation that may lead to the condition known as uremia. Kidney disease may also lead to hypertension (high blood pressure). This happens when the kidneys release a chemical called renin into the blood. Renin, in turn, helps to bring about the formation of another chemical, angiotensin. Angiotensin is a very strong blood vessel constrictor, which is instrumental in the raising of the blood pressure.

> When you eat animal flesh, you take into your system the waste products of that animal. Consequently, your kidneys not only have to take care of the waste that occurs naturally in your body, but they must also have the additional task of having to deal with the added waste products of the animal you ate.

Glomerulonephritis, inflammation of the glomeruli of the kidney, is the result of an immune response. A typical case would involve bacteria and antibodies to the bacteria coming together and forming an immune complex. These immune complexes then become entrapped in the capillaries that form the glomeruli of the kidneys. The immune complexes then bind to serum proteins called complements. Complements then attracts white blood cells, which release enzymes that destroy anything in the immediate area. This leads to inflammation of the glomeruli, which, in turn, leads to damage of the filtration membrane, thereby increasing its permeability. At this point, blood and serum proteins pass into the tubules and ultimately into the urine. This results in a drop in the osmotic pressure of the blood, which leads to increased fluid in the tissue spaces, resulting in edema. Glomerulosclerosis, fibrosis, and scarring, which results in aging of the renal glomeruli, has been demonstrated to occur in animals that were fed diets high in cholesterol or saturated fats. Hyperlipidemia, elevated lipids in the plasma, which was induced by diet, has been shown in animals to be associated with albuminuria as well as the accelerated development of glomerulosclerosis. Studies have shown accelerated glomerular damage in animals fed diets rich in cholesterol with or without saturated fats. For instance, high cholesterol intake in guinea pigs caused hypercholesterolemia (excess cholesterol in the blood) and the deposition of lipid in the glomeruli. Subsequently progressive glomerular stress injury resulted.

Hemolytic Uremic Syndrome (HUS)

Post-diarrheal Hemolytic Uremic Syndrome (D+HUS) is a severe, life-threatening condition. This potentially fatal disease has been associated with the bacteria Escherichia coli 0157:H7 (E. coli 0157:H7). It occurs in about 10 percent of those infected with E. coli O157:H7 or some other Shiga toxin-producing E. coli. Although D+HUS had been known for several decades, it was not known to be secondary to E. coli infections until 1982. It is now recognized as the most common cause of acute kidney failure in infants and young children. HUS is more common in children under the age of four than in any other group. There are more than 20,000 cases of HUS reported each year, along with 500 deaths. There was an outbreak of HUS in Japan that affected 10,000 people and killed eleven. Scotland also had an outbreak in which 400 cases were reported as well as twenty deaths.

E. coli 0157:H7 is found in the intestines of cattle and is found in milk. A study conducted to determine the presence of bacteria in milk examined bulk tank milk from 131 dairy herds in eastern South Dakota and western Minnesota for coliform and non-coliform bacteria. Coliforms were detected in 62.3 percent of bulk tank milk samples. Non-coliform bacteria were observed in 76.3 percent of bulk tank milk.[121] In another study, USDA researchers documented the presence of fecal bacteria (coliform bacteria) in milk of refrigerated trucks. They tested 861 bulk trucks in twenty-one states. Coliform bacteria were found in 95 percent of the milk samples![122]

Most bacterial infections require millions of bacteria to cause problems. However, less than a dozen E. coli 0157:H7 can cause infection. Once these E. coli enter the intestines, they begin to multiply rapidly and cling to the cells that line the intestine. The toxin (Shiga toxin) enters the cytoplasm of the cell, where it effectively takes over the cell's protein synthesis mechanism. This results in the death or serious injury to the cell. This then leads to the activation of blood platelets and the initiation of the coagulation cascade. This state of inflammation leads to the formation of clots and is the cause of bloody diarrhea. This is known as the prodromal phase of HUS. This process also occurs in the kidneys. The toxin of E. coli then enters into the general circulation of the body and attaches to white blood cells that are then carried to the kidneys. Additionally, the toxin destroys red blood cells. When the blood vessels of the kidneys are destroyed (HUS), kidney failure is inevitable. Young children and the elderly are most at risk. The elderly also face the prospect of thrombocytopenia purpura (leaking blood vessels), which can lead to a coma even death. It is during the prodromal stage of HUS that patients will often be misdiagnosed as having ulcerative colitis or appendicitis due to the inflamed intestine. Appendicitis is often thought to be the case because the pain that results from the inflamed intestine is often in the same area that is associated with the pain that is classic with appendicitis. Ulcerative colitis is often the diagnosis due to the visualization of inflammation and ulceration of the colon when a colonoscopy is performed or the presence of a thickened and inflamed colon seen on a CT scan. It is the multiple days of bloody diarrhea, low platelet count, hemolytic anemia, and acute renal failure that have come to be the definitive diagnosis of HUS.

---

121 BM Jayarao and L Wang, "A Study on the Prevalence of Gram-Negative Bacteria in Bulk Tank Milk," *Journal of Dairy Science* 82, no. 12 (December 1999): 2620–2624, https://1ref.us/1zp (accessed June 2, 2022).
122 J Van Kessel et al., "Prevalence of Salmonellae, Listeria Monocytogenes and Fecal Coliforms In Bulk Tank Milk on US Dairies," *Journal of Dairy Science*, September 2004, 2822–2830, https://1ref.us/1zq (accessed June 2, 2022).

Generally, infection of E. coli 0157:H7 results in the injury of cells that line blood vessels. As a consequence, the damage that is seen in the intestine and kidneys can also happen in other organs of the body such as the brain and pancreas.

Kidney Stones

Salts that are in the urine form kidney stones. These salts cause stones by forming a residue rather than staying dissolved in the urine. Some kidney stones result from the metabolism of proteins. One kidney stone, in particular, is the result of a high concentration of uric acid, namely the uric acid stone. Another type of kidney stone, the cystine stone, occurs due in part to the excretion of the amino acid cystine. Proteins are broken down into amino acids. If we take in too much protein, there is a resultant increase in nitrogenous wastes and ammonia, which can lead to the formation of urea and uric acid. This is in addition to the uric acid and urea, which are already present in meat.

Many kidney stones are small enough to pass through your system without you even noticing it. However, there can be problems, depending upon the size and number of the stones present. The stone can prevent the flow of urine and increase the chance of infection by clogging the ureter. They can also damage the walls of the urinary tract as they attempt to pass out of your system. In many cases there is a great deal of pain associated with the passing of larger kidney stones as they attempt to pass out of the system. Some stones are so large that surgery must be performed in order to remove them.

Generally, the amount of uric acid the body excretes is related to the amount of proteins and purines you consume. This is one reason why those with kidney stones and those without the symptoms of kidney stones would do well to lower the amount of protein in their diet to help reduce the amount of uric acid in the urine.

Gout

Gout is the result of uric acid becoming solid and forming crystals that deposit in the joints. Gout resembles many forms of arthritis. The most common site of gout is the forefoot. Gout may also affect the hand, wrist, elbow, spine, knees, ankles, hips, and shoulders. The earlier stages of gout involve soft tissue swelling. In the later stages of gout, lesions form that effectively alter the joints.

Again, here is another disease in which uric acid is involved. As such, those suffering from gout would probably do well to lower the amount of uric acid resulting from dietary intake.

Lactose Intolerance

Genetic makeup plays a factor in lactose intolerance. Caucasians generally tend not to develop lactose intolerance. Interestingly, lactose intolerance is quite common among people from Asia, Africa, the Middle East, and some Mediterranean countries, as well as among Australian Aborigines. Up to 5 percent of Caucasians and up to 75 percent of non-Caucasians living in Australia are lactose intolerant.

Many Australian babies are unnecessarily weaned because their irritability is wrongly assumed to be lactose intolerance. In reality, the severe form of this condition—known as primary lactose intolerance (where the infant does not produce lactase from birth)—is rare. Secondary lactose intolerance develops after weaning.

Blacks tend to be notoriously lactose intolerant. Moreover, the darker the person is, the more likely they are lactose intolerant. That being said, why does the government insist on giving milk to black children in school lunch programs and other social programs? If the milk causes these children to experience gastrointestinal discomfort, and the allergens in milk lead to them having increased asthma attacks, it is not much of a stretch to see why many black children do not do well in school. Can you imagine taking an exam with an upset stomach and difficulty breathing???

Why then is it that people who are allergic to milk can consume cheese and yogurt without a problem? When milk is converted to yogurt, the bacteria break down the lactose into glucose and galactose. The same thing happens with cheese. Much of the lactose is converted into the simple sugars glucose and galactose, which are much more likely to be tolerated than lactose.

Percentage of Ethnic Group with Lactose Deficiency

African Blacks 95–100
Indians 90–100

Asians 90–95
Native Americans 70–90
Mexican Americans 70–80
African Americans 70–75
Mediterranean Peoples 60–75
North American Whites 10–15
Northern Europeans 5–10

Multiple Scleroris (MS)

German scientists have determined that milk proteins produce a reaction in the myelin sheath of nerve fibers that can result in MS. Other studies have also linked dairy products to multiple sclerosis.

Acromegaly

There is a controversy brewing over a substance called IGF-I. Insulin-like growth factor I (IGF-I) is found in humans as well as in cattle. Its role is that of mediating the effects of growth hormones. BGH stimulates production of IGH-I in cows. The problem is that IGH-I can end up in the milk. Humans can then drink the milk containing the IGH-I. IGH-I can survive the trip through the digestive tract and stimulate cells in the intestine. Another problem is that high levels of IGH-I in humans lead to a disease condition known as acromegaly. Acromegaly is associated with chronic excessive levels of growth hormone that leads to giantism. It is a slowly progressive disease that may lead to death due to diabetes mellitus and hypertension. Once again, the consumer is at an impasse as to who and what to believe.

When you hear all of the propaganda about BGH being safe, you must remember that the dairy lobby has a tremendous amount of influence on the FDA. The dairy industry lobbies effectively to keep our government spending millions upon millions of dollars each year to subsidize the production of milk—milk that is not needed but is, in fact, wasted. This leads to lower milk prices, which in turn forces the small farmer out of business. As a consequence, millions more are spent by our government each year to store the incredible senseless surplus milk in the form of unsold butter, cheese, and nonfat dried milk, only to have to finally give it away via various government programs. Why are so many of our tax dollars being wasted in producing, storing, and giving away such a useless product???

Microorganisms

Milk is an ideal medium for many microorganisms.

Certain leukemia viruses (approximately 80 percent of the dairy cows in the U.S. are infected with the Bovine Leukemia Virus), the herpes simplex virus, sarcoma virus, Listeria monocytogenes, Yersinia enterocolitica, and several others are resistant to the pasteurization process milk undergoes. Some of the deadliest outbreaks of food poisoning in this country have involved pasteurized milk! In 1982, approximately 15,000 people in the state of Tennessee and nearby states fell victim to an outbreak of food poisoning caused by the bacteria Yersinia enterocolitic from pasteurized milk. In 1985, there were approximately 200,000 people in six states who fell victim to the largest outbreak of salmonella in the U.S. The culprit was pasteurized milk that was traced to a milk processing plant in the state of Illinois.

Meningitis

The bacterium E. sakasakii has been associated with cases of meningitis. This bacterium survives the pasteurization process and, therefore will be found in milk and milk products, including milk-based infant formulas!

Brucellosis

This disease affects cows, sheep, hogs, and goats, causing them to abort. With cows, even though they may have a tendency to abort and pass on a substantial number of bacilli causing the disease in their milk, they still appear to be healthy. Brucellosis can be passed on to humans and manifests itself in the form of Mediterranean Disease or Undulant fever. There are several types of brucella that affect humans: Brucella melintensis that occurs in sheep and goats, Brucella abortus that occurs in cows, and Brucella suis that occurs in hogs. All of these types of brucella can affect humans and cause them to have undulant fever. Localized brucellosis manifests itself in pulmonary disease, genitourinary disease, neurologic disease, and cardiovascular disease. If pregnant women contract brucellosis, they may abort spontaneously. A brucellosis infection is often not detected because rarely is it searched for; hence it is prone to be misdiagnosed. Symptoms include chronic fatigue, headaches, and arthritic pain. Once infected with Brucellosis, the organism can hide in the human body for years without expression.

Salmonellosis

There are over 2,300 serotypes of salmonella. Some attack only humans, some attack only animals, and others attack both humans and animals. Salmonellosis is transmitted only by the anal-oral route. In other words, the bacteria responsible for salmonellosis is found in the feces of humans and animals that results in infection when ingested. Hence, one should be genuinely concerned about food handlers and their personal hygiene since they play a significant role in unwittingly placing bacteria into food. Humans can become infected with salmonella by eating contaminated beef, pork, chicken, turkey, and dairy products. Salmonella can survive the pasteurization process. Salmonella can remain viable in butter for up to nine months! Butter readily supports growth of salmonella at room temperature, but refrigeration or freezing for brief periods does not eliminate it. This can readily lead to outbreaks. One such outbreak occurred in Chicago and caused 150,000 people to fall ill. Published reports of outbreaks tend to be rare because the outbreaks may not be recognized for several reasons. Milk is an extremely common food item, which makes reporting exposure to milk unlikely, obscuring an association. Typhimurium is one of the most common serotypes of Salmonella, making the detection of outbreaks more difficult in the absence of subtyping. Cooking often destroys some salmonella that may be present in the meat. However, when meats are allowed to sit out in the open at room temperature for extended periods of time, the remaining salmonella will reproduce rapidly. Infection by salmonella can cause several distinct stages of disease, namely enterecolitis (gastroenteritis), enteric fever, bacteremia, focal infection, and chronic carrier state.

Enterocolitis (gastroenteritis) may occur in as little as six or as late as seventy-two hours after eating food contaminated with salmonella. This will usually involve nausea and vomiting followed by diarrhea, constipation, muscle aches and pain, abdominal pain, and cramps.

Enteric fever (typhoid fever) has an incubation period usually of ten to fourteen days and may vary from seven to twenty-one days. Abdominal complications such as intestinal perforation and intestinal hemorrhage may result. In addition, other complications such as meningitis, endocarditis, arthritis, osteomyelitis, pneumonia, bone marrow suppression, and parotitis may result as well. Bacteremia (bacteria in the blood) may last for days or weeks. Focal infections (soft tissues, benign tumors, malignant tumors) are expressed in endocarditis, pericarditis, appendicitis, cholecystitis, salpingitis, intra-abdominal abscesses, pneumonia, mycotic aneurysm, urinary tract infection, bone and joint infection, and meningitis.

As if the foregoing phenomena were not enough, the victim of salmonellosis will be in a chronic carrier state. Simply put, the victim will excrete salmonella for more than a year!!! The number of cases of salmonellosis is on the increase. In 1998, 43,700 cases of salmonellosis were reported. It is estimated that there are between 2,000,000 to 4,000,000 cases of salmonella in the U.S. alone each year because for every case that is reported, ten to 100 cases go unreported. In addition, approximately 1,000 to 2,000 people die in the U.S. from salmonella every year.

The newest member of the salmonella family that is causing great concern is Salmonella typhimurium DT 104. It has made its mark in Europe and is now in the U.S. The concern of Salmonella typhimurium DT 104 centers on its resistance to antibiotics. It has been discovered that bacteria carry genes with antibiotic resistance. These genes are often found on plasmids. Plasmids are extrachromosomal self-replicating structures that carry genes for a variety of functions not essential for cell growth. Scientists have found that the genes responsible for antibiotic resistance in Salmonella typhimurium DT 104 are right on the chromosome, which makes it easier to pass antibiotic resistance along to the next generation. Salmonella typhimurium DT 104 has proven resistant to the major classes of antibiotics and even shows resistance to the latest powerful class of antibiotics called fluoroquinolones.

Scientists from the University of Minnesota tested cattle from 110 organic and conventional dairy farms in Minnesota, Wisconsin, Michigan, and New York. They acquired 22,417 fecal samples and 4,570 samples from the farm environment. Salmonella was detected n 4.8 percent of the fecal samples and 5.9 percent of the environmental samples. Perhaps most disturbing was the fact that 92.7 percent of the dairies had at least one Salmonella-positive sample.[123]

Klebsiella

Klebsiella is a rod-shaped bacterium that is heat resistant and therefore can easily survive pasteurization. Klebsiella causes respiratory infection such as bronchitis but is known to cause pneumonia. Klebsiella pneumonia is more serious because it forms abscesses (pus pockets) in the lung and destroys lung tissue. Hence, klebsiella pneumonia has a high mortality rate.

Botulism

Botulism is a dangerous and often fatal disease. The toxins involved prevent nerve endings from liberating an important chemical substance, acetylcholine, which is necessary for nerve impulses. Since the toxins prevent the liberation of acetylcholine, death results from the paralysis of muscles controlling breathing.

Botulism is caused by the neurotoxins produced by the little demons named clostridium botulinum. There are several distinct toxins produced by clostridium botulinum, types A, B, C, D, E, F, and G. Types A, B, E, and F have been shown to cause disease in humans. Types C and D have been shown to cause disease in animals.

Foods contaminated with the toxins produced by clostridium botulinum often appear and taste normal. If you eat even a very small sample of contaminated food, there will be more than enough toxins in it to cause a serious episode of botulism. Less than 1/100,000 of a gram is needed to kill a mouse. This amount can barely be seen with an unaided eye.

> Botulism is caused by the neurotoxins produced by the little demons named clostridium botulinum.

Generally, within a twelve-hour period after eating contaminated food, the toxin begins to affect the nervous system. Diplopia (double vision),

---

123 Charles Fossler et al., "Prevalence of Salmonella spp on Conventional and Organic Dairy Farms," *Journal of the American Veterinary Medical Association* 225, no. 4 (August 2004): 567–573, https://1ref.us/1zr (accessed June 2, 2022).

blurred vision, and vertigo appear first. This is followed by difficulty in breathing and swallowing. If the amount of toxin is large, slurred speech will then occur, followed by respiratory failure that leads to death if an antitoxin is not administered in time.

Listeria Monocytogenes

Listeria monocytogenes is the culprit of the disease Listeriosis. This disease has two primary syndromes, an invasive form and noninvasive form of the illness. The invasive form of the illness is characterized by a sudden onset of severe symptoms, such as meningitis, septicemia, primary bacteremia, endocarditis, flu-like symptoms, i.e., fever, vomiting, diarrhea, and chills. The noninvasive form of this disease is characterized by fever and gastroenteritis.

Listeria infections result in hospitalization rates 4.5 times that of Salmonella infections, higher than any other pathogen, and resulted in approximately half of all reported deaths from food-borne pathogens.

Milk is an ideal medium for bacteria and a host of viruses. Pathogenic bacteria are passed to humans through milk and milk products. We are led to believe that the pasteurization process renders milk safe to consume because it destroys injurious bacteria and other organisms. Listeria can easily survive the pasteurization process. A study was performed at the University of Wisconsin showing the effect of pasteurization on the microorganism listeria monocytogens. In the study cows were inoculated with listeria. The milk from these cows was then pooled for two to four days and then heated to the standard minimum high-temperature, short-time treatment (162 degrees Fahrenheit for sixteen seconds) required by the U.S. FDA for pasteurizing milk. In eleven of the twelve pasteurization trials, live listeria bacteria was successfully isolated from the milk after heat treatment.[124] Simply stated, this study demonstrated the ability of listeria to survive the pasteurization process. These listeria will still be able to grow during refrigeration and be consumed by the unknowing public.

---

124 MP Doyle et al., "Survival of Listeria Monocytogenes In Milk During High-Temperature, Short-Time Pasteurization," *Applied and Environmental Microbiology* 53, no. 7 (July 1987): 1433–1438, https://1ref.us/1zs (accessed June 2, 2022).

Campylobacter

Campylobacter jejuni is the culprit responsible for Campylobateriosis, the leading cause of bacterial infections in food-borne illnesses in the U.S. What is quite disturbing is the recent discovery that campylobacter can lead to a disease called Guillain-Barré syndrome. Guillain-Barré syndrome is an autoimmune disease characterized by fever, neuromuscular paralysis, and inflammation of many nerves at once. It begins with an abnormal sensation of the feet, followed by paralysis and weakness of the legs; it then ascends to the arms, trunk, and face. Approximately 50 percent of patients with Guillain-Barré syndrome have evidence of recent Campylobacter infection at the onset of neurologic symptoms. In addition, Campylobacter infection appears to be involved in Reiter syndrome, a condition marked by inflammation of the urethra, conjunctivitis, and arthritis.[125]

Enterohemorrhagic Escherichia coli

Escherichia coli bacteria are normal harmless residents of the digestive tract of animals and humans. However, there are groups of E. coli that can cause disease. One of the most dangerous serotypes is 0157:H7.

Hemorrhagic colitis (bleeding colon) is a principal manifestation of infection with enterohemorrhagic E. coli. This is characterized by bloody diarrhea, vomiting, and abdominal cramps. This may last from a couple of days to a little over a week. A small percentage, 3–7 percent, of these cases may progress to hemolytic uremic syndrome and thrombotic thrombocytopenic purpura.

Tyrotoxicosis

This potentially fatal condition results from the ingestion of tyrotoxin, which can be found in stale milk, cheese, and ice cream. It is marked by vertigo, headache, vomiting, chills, muscular cramps, extreme exhaustion, and death.

---

125 I Nachamki, BM Allos, T Ho, "Campylobacter Species and Guillain-Barré Syndrome," *Clinical Microbiology Reviews* 11, no. 3 (July 1998): 555–567, https://1ref.us/1zt (accessed June 2, 2022).

Hypervitaminosis D

Another way that the dairy industry encourages us to buy milk is to tell us that we need vitamin D and that milk is an excellent source of vitamin D. How nice! We are told that milk contains vitamin D as well as calcium. Actually, calcium needs vitamin D to react with it in order to be of any value. The government has set the amount of vitamin D in milk to be 400 IU per quart. The original purpose for vitamin D was to eliminate the disease called rickets. A growing problem is the actual amount of vitamin D in milk. Studies have been done which show too much and too little vitamin D in milk. If there is too much vitamin D in milk, it can lead to a condition known as hypervitaminosis D.

Antibiotics

Many people think that milk is a pure and natural food. This way of thinking was challenged by the Wall Street Journal when it launched an independent investigation of milk in ten different cities. Roughly 40 percent of the samples had detectable drug residues. This should be of great concern, especially since seventy-five or more drugs are given to dairy cows in an attempt to prevent/cure a variety of illnesses. In addition, this should be of great concern to everybody because of the allergic reactions that are likely to occur in people who drink milk with antibiotic residues. Of greater concern is the likelihood of creating new breeds of microorganisms called "superbugs" that are resistant to the antibiotics that are in use today.

Excess Protein

Milk is high in fat. To avoid the fat in milk, many people have switched to low-fat and non-fat milk. This may address the problem of fat; however, another problem is created. These types of milk have higher amounts of protein. The higher amounts of protein can lead to osteoporosis, allergic reactions, and kidney problems.

Fat

Milk is high in fat. Excessive fat in the diet can lead to atherosclerosis and is implicated in breast as well as colon cancer. In addition, the high fat content of milk raises the issue of a higher concentration of pesticides and other harmful fat-soluble chemicals the cow may have ingested.

Milk is also rich in a substance called xanthine oxidase. Xanthine oxidase has been implicated in playing a role in artery disease by lessening the amount of phospholipids in the heart and arteries.

Calcium

As with protein, the problem is not that we are getting enough calcium; the real problem is that we are getting too much calcium! Try finding a case in the medical literature of someone being calcium deficient! Excess calcium can get into your muscles, causing them to contract needlessly. It can also get into the joints where it can cause arthritis. Perhaps most disturbing is that excess calcium can be deposited in the arteries where it can contribute to arteriosclerosis and calcification.

Drinking raw milk is not the answer!!!

In order to avoid the hazards of commercial pasteurized milk, there are people who want to go "natural" in order to get the vitamins, enzymes, minerals, nutrients, etc., they have been led to believe they need, in a natural state, so they purchase raw cow's milk! This author is of the belief that the argument between pasteurized milk and raw milk is akin to debating the virtues of pasteurized sewage versus raw sewage. No matter how you try to shape the argument or promote the product, cow's milk was designed for baby cows and not humans of any age.

Raw milk advocates often point to the so-called fact that humans have been consuming raw milk for centuries. However, they conveniently fail to see that this argument goes nowhere because people have been doing all types of things for centuries. Longevity of a practice is not a criterion for healthfulness of the practice. Moreover, the milk of the past was not from antibiotic-, growth- hormone-, pesticide-, herbicide-, cancer-, BLV-, BIV-, and BSE-laden cows!

All of the benefits that raw milk advocates trumpet may seem "safe" because raw milk is viewed as a "live" food as opposed to pasteurized milk, which is viewed as a dead food. Raw milk advocates believe that the "competitive flora" (bacteria from the gut), enzymes, and particles from the immune system of a cow, make raw milk safe. However, raw milk can be quite dangerous! How dangerous? If raw milk was such a safe food, how is it that many infections are passed onto the suckling calf from milk containing infectious agents? BLV, BSE, BIV are passed from the mother to its suckling calf. If over half of the states in this country do not allow the sale of raw milk and the FDA does not allow it to be shipped between states for consumer use, that should tell you something! Since raw milk does not undergo pasteurization to kill bacteria and viruses, untold numbers of them are allowed to roam freely in raw milk, ready to be ingested into the stomach of some unsuspecting consumer! Raw milk is known to contain the bacteria Coviella burnetti which is the causative agent in Q fever, E. coli O157:H7 that is the same organism that was responsible for the food poisoning outbreak in the northwestern U.S., Salmonella, Listeria, M. tuberculosis, staphylococcus, and Yersinia. These organisms can cause anything from nausea to death. Campylobacter outbreaks are common, and the organism can be found in apparently healthy cattle.

If people are intent on consuming raw milk filled with pus, feces, BSE, BIV, BLV, E. coli, salmonella, etc., etc., there is no amount of data that can change their minds. Therefore, for those of you who are open in your thinking regarding milk and raw milk, I hope that you will take the pages of this book to heart.

Milk and Fertility

Milk contains high levels of estrogens and other hormones. When these hormones are consumed in high quantities, a man's sperm count can be affected negatively. Total dairy food intake was inversely related to sperm morphology. Compared with men in the lowest quartile of total dairy food intake (0–1.65 servings/day), normal sperm morphology (95 percent confidence intervals) was 1.5 percent (−0.3 to 3.3), 2.7 percent (0.9 to 4.5), and 3.0 percent (1.0 to 4.9) lower for men in the second, third, and highest quartiles of intake, respectively (4.33 to 13.26 servings/day for men in the highest quartile). In addition, there was a suggestion of an inverse association between total dairy intake and total sperm count and sperm concentration.[126]

---

126 M Afeiche et al., "Dairy Food Intake In Relation to Semen Quality and Reproductive Hormone Levels Among Physically Active Young Men," *Human Reproduction* 28, no. 8 (August 2013): 2265–2275, https://1ref.us/1zu (accessed June 2, 2022).

Dietary galactose may adversely affect ovarian function. Beta-galactosidase (lactase) causes the breakdown of lactose and its component sugars, galactose and glucose. Hypolactasia, or the decreased amount of lactase present in the body for the digestion of lactose, is a common occurrence in the world, especially after infancy when nursing ceases. Those individuals who have high levels of lactase as well as high levels of milk consumption will have greater dietary exposure to galactose. There is sufficient evidence that galactose may be toxic to ovarian germ cells. It has been found that fertility at older ages is lower, and the decline in fertility with aging is steeper in populations with high per capita consumption of milk and greater ability to digest its lactose component. Dietary galactose may deleteriously affect ovarian function.[127]

---

127 DW Cramer, H Xu, T Sahi, "Adult Hypolactasia, Milk Consumption, and Age-Specific Fertility," *American Journal of Epidemiology* 139, no. 3 (February 1994): 282–289, https://1ref.us/1zv (accessed June 2, 2022).

Chapter 8

DECREASE YOUR CANCER RISK!

There is a unique growth hormone that is found in humans, and it is arguably THE most potent growth hormone in humans. Interestingly, this same hormone is found in the milk of cows. The hormones are nearly identical. This becomes problematic when humans consume milk from cows because of the increased amount of this hormone, IGF-1, that begins to flow in the blood, thereby increasing its serum levels. The issue becomes one of effect. Given that IGF-1 is a powerful growth stimulator for normal cells, one can't help but reason that it would be involved in accelerating the growth of tumors and, ultimately, cancer cells. IGF-1 has been implicated in a number of cancers; however, as usual, there is much scientific debate concerning IGF-1 and its role in cancer. Part of the problem is that milk is a very complex fluid with numerous hormones at various concentrations. Consequently, studying IGF-1 in isolation is likely to give a different result than studying IGF-1 in milk in its natural state.

Studies have shown that drinking milk does increase serum IGF-1 levels.[128] Modern dairy technology has made dairy products an abundant source of this growth stimulant. Since 1985, U.S. dairy farmers have been allowed to inject cows with recombinant bovine growth hormone (rbGH aka rBST), a genetically engineered bovine growth hormone developed by the chemical giant Monsanto. RbGH was designed to increase milk production. One of the side effects of the increased milk production is

---

128 E Giovannucci, M Pollak, Y Liu, et al. "Nutritional Predictors of Insulin-like Growth Factor I and Their Relationships to Cancer in Men," *Cancer Epidemiol Biomarkers and Prevention* 12, no. 2 (2003): 84–89.

an increase in IGF-1 in the milk.[129][130] Since IGF-1 is not destroyed by pasteurization, the overall effect is that milk appears to raise IGF-1 levels in humans.

However, there is more to cancer promotion by dairy foods than IGF-1. Most dairy products are high in saturated fat—and fat is the number one suspect when it comes to the cause of most common cancers in Western societies. Recent studies have linked lactose, the sugar in milk, and fat in milk with ovarian cancer. Calcium in milk works to lower concentrations of a specific form of vitamin D that protects against prostate cancer, thereby raising men's overall risk. Cows are milked while they are pregnant. Consequently, during this time, cows secrete high levels of estrogen into their milk. Therefore, by consuming cow's milk, one is also consuming inordinate amounts of hormones. The hormones in milk, specifically estrogens, are involved in cancers of the reproductive organs. The resulting increase in hormones in the body causes a number of hormone-dependent problems, ranging from early onset of menstruation to PMS and fibroids.

Breast Cancer

Breast cancer hits home for me. I have had several close friends die from breast cancer. I remember well the night one dear friend, overwhelmed with the thought she had breast cancer, allowed me to feel the lump. She was frightened with the prospect of her demise. Sadly, the disease claimed her as a victim. It was sad beyond words to see a beautiful woman in the summer of her life succumb to a disease that took her beautiful frame and left her with just skin and bones.

There are two main types of breast cancer, Ductal carcinoma and Lobular carcinoma. Ductal carcinoma, the most common form of breast cancer, begins in the ducts that move milk from the breast to the nipple. Lobular carcinoma begins in the lobules, the structures that are responsible for making milk. Lobular breast cancer rates are on the rise.[131]

---

129 "Recombinant Bovine Growth Hormone," American Cancer Society, https://1ref. us/1zw (accessed June 6, 2022).

130 J Beasley et al., "Associations of Serum Insulin-like Growth Factor-I and Insulin-like Growth Factor-binding Protein," *The British Journal of Nutrition* 111, no. 5 (March 2014): 847–853, https://1ref.us/1zx (accessed June 6, 2022).

131 Veronica Hackethal, "New Study Suggests Milk Could Increase Breast Cancer Risk," Medscape, February 28, 2020, https://1ref.us/1zy (accessed June 6, 2022).

Breast cancer statistics are a growing concern. As of January 2020, there are more than 3.5 million women with a history of breast cancer in the U.S. This includes women currently being treated and women who have finished treatment. About 12 percent of women will develop invasive breast cancer during their lifetime. In 2020, it was estimated that 276,480 new cases of invasive breast cancer will be diagnosed in women in the U.S., along with 48,530 new cases of non-invasive (in situ) breast cancer. Though women get most of the attention when it comes to breast cancer, men develop breast cancer as well. It was anticipated that nearly 2,620 new cases of invasive breast cancer will be diagnosed in men in 2020. The lifetime risk of breast cancer for men is about 1 in 883. Approximately 42,170 women in the U.S. are expected to die in 2020 from breast cancer. Fortunately, death rates have been steady in women under fifty since 2007 but have continued to drop in women over fifty. There has been a drop in the overall death rate from breast cancer by 1.3 percent per year from 2013 to 2017. The death rate from breast cancer for women in the U.S. is second only to lung cancer.[132]

Cow's milk contains nutrients and anabolic hormones that lead to an explosive growth that is natural for cows but not for humans. As a result, and not surprisingly, the consumption of cow's milk by humans promotes growth, and such growth has been linked to an increased risk of breast cancer. Gary E. Fraser, MBChB, Ph.D., noted that the study gives "fairly strong evidence that either dairy milk or some other factor closely related to drinking dairy milk is a cause of breast cancer in women. "Consuming as little as 1/4 to 1/3 cup of dairy milk per day was associated with an increased risk of breast cancer of 30%," Fraser said. "By drinking up to one cup per day, the associated risk went up to 50%, and for those drinking two to three cups per day, the risk increased further to 70% to 80%."[133]

A study of 1,893 women diagnosed with early-stage invasive breast cancer revealed that eating more high-fat dairy products was linked to higher death rates. As little as half a serving per day increased risk significantly. Since hormones are stored in fat, consuming high fat, rather than low-fat, dairy products likely means women are consuming more

---

132 "Breast Cancer Statistics," Breastcancer.org, https://1ref.us/1zz (accessed June 6, 2022).
133 "Milk and Cheese Increase Risk for Breast Cancer," Physicians Committee for Responsible Medicine, https://1ref.us/200 (accessed June 6, 2022).

estrogen.[134] A second large study of 1,941 women found that women who consumed the highest amounts of cheddar, American, and cream cheeses had a 53 percent higher risk for breast cancer.[135]

A study conducted by researchers at the National Cancer Institute assayed milk in grocery stores for fifteen estrogens, including estradiol and estrone, along with thirteen metabolic derivatives of these female hormones. They found that whole milk contained the smallest amount of estrogens with skim milk and buttermilk with the highest quantities.[136] This should come as no surprise since pregnant cows produce numerous hormones, some of which tell their own mammary tissues to grow. The researchers showed that the mélange of estrogens varies considerably between milks. Whole milk contained the smallest quantity of estrogens, and amounts ascended from 2 percent to skim and buttermilk. In all of these milks tested, the majority of estrogens had undergone some minor chemical modification that rendered them less directly bioavailable and less hormonally active. However, though modified, these modified, or conjugated, estrogens were not rendered inert. The conversion of these estrogens was such that they could be converted back to their more potent parent compounds. The NCI scientists noted that studies by others have shown that relative to free, bioavailable estrogens, conjugated ones take longer to get from the gut into the blood Additionally, conjugated estrogens found in milk are likely to have longer half-lives than non-conjugated estrogens due to first pass metabolism in the liver.[137]

When it comes to environmental factors and breast cancer, the role of the bovine leukemia virus (BLV) cannot be ignored. The bovine leukemia virus, BLV, is a cancer-causing virus, and it is estimated that 84 percent of dairy herds in the United States are infected.[138] Older cows are more

---

134 CH Kroenke, ML Kwan, C Sweeney, A Castillo, BJ Caan, "High- and Low-fat Dairy Intake, Recurrence, and Mortality after Breast Cancer Diagnosis," *Journal of the National Cancer Institute* 105, no. 9 (May 2013): 616–623, https://1ref.us/201 (accessed June 6, 2022).
135 D Farlow, X Xu, T. Veenstra, "Quantitative Measurement of Endogenous Estrogen Metabolites, Risk-factors for Development of Breast Cancer, In Commercial Milk Products by LC-MS/MS, *Journal of Chromatography* 877, no. 13 (May 2009): 1327–1334, https://1ref.us/202 (accessed June 6, 2022).
136 M Frie et al., "Dairy Cows Naturally Affected with Bovine Leukemia Virus Exhibit Abnormal B- and T-Cell Phenotypes," *Frontiers In Veterinary Science* (July 14, 2017), https://1ref.us/203 (accessed June 6, 2022).
137 Frie, "Dairy Cows."
138 G Buehring et al., "Bovine Leukemia Virus DNA in Human Breast Tissue," *Emerging Infectious Diseases* 20, no. 5 (2014): 772–782, https://1ref.us/204 (accessed June 6, 2022).

likely to be infected than younger cows given the time it takes the disease to take hold. For example, 30 percent of first-lactation cows were infected versus 59 percent of fourth or greater lactation cows. This is a worldwide phenomenon—Japan, Canada, South America, China, and many other countries are reporting BLV prevalence similar to the U.S.

BLV is of concern to humans because it can cross the placenta of a cow and can be found in the milk of an infected cow.[139] Additionally, BLV has been found in human blood.[140] In the 1970s, studies were launched to determine to what extent, if any, the role of animal products, specifically from cattle, might play in the infection of humans. Using the testing methods of the time, no antibodies to BLV were detected in human serum samples in these studies. This led scientists to safely conclude that there was no evidence that BLV was capable of infecting humans. However, in 2003, Dr. Gertrude Buehring and her team at the School of Public Health, University of California, Berkeley, re-examined the issue. Instead of using the same equipment that was used previously in the 1970s, they used modern immunological techniques that were about 100 times more sensitive than those used in the 1970s.[141] The researchers found that 39 percent of 257 human serum samples tested had antibodies against the BLV p24 capsid antigen which indicated exposure to BLV antigen, but not necessarily infection with BLV. In 2014, Dr. Gertrude Buehring and her team of researchers examined 219 human breast tissue samples for the presence of BLV DNA and showed that 44 percent were positive.[142] Moreover, the researchers demonstrated that the viral DNA was confined to the secretory mammary epithelial cells and that 6 percent were positive for BLV p24 capsid protein. These observations in the study indicate that the virus may be replicating in some humans.

---

139 Y Sajiki et al., "Intrauterine Infection with Bovine Leukemia Virus In Pregnant Dam with High Viral Load, *The Journal of Veterinary Medical Science* 79, no. 12 (November 2017): 2036–2039, https://1ref.us/205 (accessed June 6, 2022).

140 G Buehring et al., "Bovine Leukemia Virus Discovered In Human Blood," *BMC Infectious Diseases* 19, no. 1 (April 2019): 297, https://1ref.us/206 (accessed June 6, 2022).

141 G Buehring, S Philpott, K Choi, "Humans Have Antibodies Reactive with Bovine Leukemia Virus," *AIDS Research and Human Retroviruses* 19, no.12 (December 2003): 1105–1113, https://1ref.us/1y5 (accessed June 2, 2022).

142 G Buehring et al., "Bovine Leukemia Virus DNA In Human Breast Tissue," *Emerging Infectious Diseases* 20, no. 5 (May 2014): 772–782, https://1ref.us/207 (accessed June 6, 2022).

In September 2015, Buehring and colleagues reported the results of a case-control study on the association of BLV with healthy and cancerous breast tissue.[143] They examined 239 archived formalin-fixed paraffin-embedded breast tissue samples for the presence of BLV DNA in mammary epithelial cells. The 239 samples came from 114 women diagnosed with breast cancer, twenty-one with premalignant changes in breast tissue, and 104 women with neither malignant nor premalignant cells. The researchers determined that BLV DNA was present in 59 percent of breast tissues from women with breast cancer, from 38 percent of women with premalignant breast changes, and from 29 percent of normal control samples. The finding of BLV DNA in almost a third of breast tissues from normal women should be a cause of alarm given that it may take twenty to thirty years for the cancer to express itself in the form of a clinically detectable tumor.[144]

Another chemical of interest in the genesis of breast cancer is called insulin-like growth factor IGF-1. Milk is rich in naturally occurring IGF-1. The IGF-1 found in cows is identical to the IGF-1 found in humans. The levels of IGF-1 increase when one consumes milk.

Cancer of the Colon and Rectum

Cancer of the colon and rectum ranks third in incidence of new cases and death rates in the U.S.,surpassed only by lung and breast cancer in women and prostate and lung cancer in men. In2021, approximately 149,500 new cases of colon and rectal cancer were diagnosed. During this time, approximately 52,980 people died from colon and rectal cancer. In 2018, there were anestimated 1,365,135 people living with colorectal cancer in the United States.[144,145]

The incidence of colorectal cancer increases with age. It begins to rise at the age of forty and peaks at seventy-five to eighty years. Carcinoma of the rectum is more common in men, whereas carcinoma of the colon, more specifically the right colon, is more common in women. Approximately

---

143 G Buehring et al., "Exposure to Bovine Leukemia Virus Is Associated with Breast Cancer: A Case-Control Study," *PLoS One* 10, no. 9 (September 2015), https://1ref.us/208 (accessed June 6, 2022).
144 Buehring, "Exposure to Bovine Leukemia."
145 "Cancer Stat Facts: Colorectal Cancer," NIH, https://1ref.us/209 (accessed June 6, 2022).

five percent of patients have multiple synchronous colonic cancer, i.e., two or more carcinomas occurring simultaneously. Approximately 2 percent of patients have metachronous carcinomas, i.e., a new primary lesion in a patient who previously underwent a resection for cancer. The overwhelming majority, 95 percent, of malignant tumors of the colon and rectum are adenocarcinomas.

Studies now suggest that children who consume high levels of dairy products may have a greater risk of developing colorectal cancer in adulthood. From 1937 through 1939, nearly 5,000 children living in England and Scotland were involved in a study regarding family food consumption. The National Health Service Central Register was used to ascertain cancer registrations and deaths between 1948 and 2005 in the traced cohort members totaling 4,383.[146]

During the follow-up period, 770 cancer registrations or cancer deaths occurred. High childhood total dairy intake was associated with a near-tripling in the odds of colorectal cancer compared with low intake, independent of meat, fruit, and vegetable intakes and socioeconomic indicators. Milk intake showed a similar association with colorectal cancer risk.[147] The conclusion of the study showed that diet rich in dairy products during childhood is associated with a greater risk of colorectal cancer in adulthood.

Results of surgical treatment are better for those with cancer of the colon than for those with cancer of the rectum. Average five-year survival rates for colorectal cancer are 80 percent if it is limited to the bowel wall, 30 percent if there are regional nodal metastases, and 5 percent if there are distant metastases or locally unresectable tumors.

Approximately 10 percent of the lesions discovered are not able to be resected during surgery. In addition, 20 percent of patients have liver or some other distant metastases. Consequently, surgery as a cure can only be performed on about 70 percent of the patients. The surgical death rate is roughly 2–6 percent. The survival rate of patients undergoing surgery is approximately 55 percent, and the overall survival rate of all stages is about 35 percent.

---

146 J van der Pols et al., "Childhood Dairy Intake and Adult Cancer Risk: 65-y Follow-up of the Boyd Orr Cohort," *The American Journal of Clinical Nutrition* 86, no. 6 (December 2007):1722–1729, https://1ref.us/20a (accessed June 6, 2022).
147 van der Pols, "Childhood Dairy Intake."

Migrant studies have suggested an environmental factor in the susceptibility to colon cancer. Observations of Japanese migrants show that their risk for colon cancer progressively increases to the point of approximating that of whites in the U.S. Similar findings have been discovered with Poles, black Africans, and Norwegians who migrated to the U.S. The role of environmental factors is substantiated further by the variable risk within countries. There is a substantial increase in Japan with aging, especially among those with increased consumption of milk and meat products.

There is a much higher incidence of colorectal cancer in developed countries, more specifically the U.S., New Zealand, Australia, and Western Europe. Consequently, attention has been turned to diet as a key environmental factor in the etiology of colorectal cancer.

One study investigated the effects of a shift from a well-balanced mixed diet to a lacto-ovo vegetarian diet on the mutagenic activity in urine and feces. Three months after the dietary shift, the concentration of fecal direct-acting mutagens decreased significantly, although the total mutagenic activity excreted in feces per twenty-four hours was not different between the two diet periods. Both the concentration and total amount of promutagens in the urine were decreased after three months on the lacto-ovo vegetarian diet. The decrease in fecal mutagenic activity might be explained by an increased consumption of dietary fiber that leads to increased water concentration in feces, and thereby resulting in a dilution of fecal mutagenic compounds.[148]

> There is a much higher incidence of colorectal cancer in developed countries, more specifically the U.S., New Zealand, Australia, and Western Europe.

In a study of the role of diet and stool biochemistry in human colorectal carcinogens, twenty-four-hour food, urine, and stool samples were collected from a randomly selected group of individuals from two populations with a four-fold difference in colorectal cancer risk: Chinese in Shanghai, People's Republic of China (low-risk group) and Chinese-Americans of similar ages in San Francisco County (high-risk group). The findings of the study support the hypothesis that colorectal cancer

---

148 G Johansson et al. "The Effect of a Shift from a Mixed Diet to a Lacto-Vegetarian Diet on Human Urinary and Fecal Mutagenic Activity," *Carcinogenesis* 13, no. 2 (February 1992):153–157, https://1ref.us/20b (accessed June 6, 2022).

risk is increased by the consumption of high fat, high protein, and low carbohydrate diets and is associated with high levels of cholesterol in stool as well as increased daily output of 3-methyl-histidine and malonaldehyde in urine.[149]

A prospective study of 88,751 women aged thirty-four to fifty-nine without a history of cancer, inflammatory bowel disease, or familial polyposis concluded that after adjusting for total energy intake, animal fat was positively associated with the risk of colon cancer. No such association was found for vegetable fat. Fish and chicken without skin were associated with increased risk.[150]

Adenomatous colonic polyps contain neoplastic epithelium with varying degrees of dysplasia. This is evidenced by the fact that most small clusters of cancer are found within adenomatous polyps, small isolated colonic carcinomas are rarely found. Adenomatous polyps have a tendency to occur in patients who subsequently develop cancer and actually predate the cancer by ten to fifteen years. Adenomas and carcinogens appear to have in common epidemiologic and pathogenetic factors. Epidemiologic studies show that population groups with higher rates of colonic adenomas also have a tendency to be the same groups with higher rates of colon cancer.

Fat in the diet enhances cholesterol and bile acid synthesis by the liver, thereby causing the amounts of these sterols in the colon to increase. The anaerobic bacteria in the colon convert these chemicals to secondary bile acids. Secondary bile acids are promoters of carcinogens.

A diet high in animal fat may be instrumental in the origin of a bacterial flora capable of producing the chemicals azoreductase, nitro-reductase, and beta-glucuronidase, all of which have a high potential to convert bile acid and neutral sterols to carcinogens or cocarcinogens in the colon. Colonic bacteria and secondary bile acids are often implicated in the pathogenesis of cancer of the colon. The activity of fecal 7-alpha-dehydroxylase is increased in patients with colon cancer than in those

---

149 KS Yeung et al., "Comparisons of Diet and Biochemical Characteristics of Stool and Urine between Chinese Populations with Low and High Colorectal Cancer Rates," *Journal of the National Cancer Institute* 83, no. 1 –(January 1991): 46–50, https://1ref.us/20c (accessed June 6, 2022).
150 W Willett, M Stampfer, G Colditz, B Rosner, F Speizer, "Relation of Meat, Fat, and Fiber Intake to the Risk of Colon Cancer In a prospective Study Among Women," *The New England Journal of Medicine* 323, no. 24 (December 1990): 1664–1672, https://1ref.us/20d (accessed June 6, 2022).

without colon cancer. It is also important in the conversion of cholic and chenodeoxycholic acids to deoxycholic and lithocholic acids.

The role of bile acids in carcinogenesis may be that of promotion rather than of being direct carcinogens. When certain bile acids are added to specific carcinogens, an increased yield of experimentally-induced tumors results. This experiment was carried out in rodents; how this would work in humans is not certain. The yield of tumors resulting from certain carcinogenic agents is also increased when bile is detoured to the small intestine, i.e., the ileum. Therefore, it is assumed that certain bile acids may promote the development of carcinogenesis.

Short-chain fatty acids are made in the colon via bacterial fermentation of dietary fiber. Butyrate has antineoplastic effects on colon carcinoma cells that exist in humans. The ratio of butyrate production was found to be less in patients with colon cancer and adenomas compared to healthy controls.

On a less technical note, the substance sulforaphane, which is found in large amounts in broccoli, may be responsible for increasing the production of enzymes in the body's cells that fight cancer-causing agents. The vitamin folate has been implicated in preventing rectal cancer. In a study of women who ate 300 micrograms or more of folate per day, they had half the risk of rectal cancer than those who consumed less than 200 micrograms per day. Men who consumed 385 mcg or more folate per day had two-thirds the risk of rectal cancer than those who consumed less than 250 mcg per day.

Testicular Cancer

Testicular cancer is the most commonly diagnosed cancer of North American men aged fifteen to forty. Data from the Testicular Cancer Research Center shows that the number one and two countries with the highest rate of testicular cancer are Denmark and Switzerland. Denmark and Switzerland also have the highest per capita consumption of cheese in the world.

Studies have shown that high dairy, particularly cheese, intake is associated with an elevated risk of testicular cancer.[151]

---

151 M Garner et al., "Dietary Risk Factors for Testicular Carcinoma," *International Journal of Cancer* 106, no. 6 (2003): 934–941, https://1ref.us/20e (accessed June 6, 2022).

Stomach (Gastric) cancer

Stomach cancer is cancer that affects the lining of the stomach. It is estimated that in 2022, about 26,380 cases of stomach cancer would be diagnosed with nearly 60 percent more cases in men than in women: 15,900 and 10,480 respectively. About 11,090 people will die from this type of cancer (6,690 men and 4,400 women). Stomach cancer mostly affects older people. The average age of people when they are diagnosed is sixty-eight. An average of 60 percent of those diagnosed with stomach cancer each year are sixty-five or older. The risk that a man will develop stomach cancer in his lifetime is about 1 in 96.For women the chance is about 1 in 152. cancer in the U.S. Stomach cancer accounts for about 1.5% of all new cancers diagnosed in the US each year. .[152]

Research points to IGF-1 as being instrumental in the initiation and progression of stomach cancer by acting upon the receptor sites of the cells and thereby altering their function. IGF-1 has also been implicated in tumor angiogenesis (the making of blood vessels for the tumor).[153]

Pancreatic Cancer

The American Cancer Society estimates that in 2022, pancreatic cancer in the United Stateswould be diagnosed in about 62,210 people (32,970 men and 29,240 women). It is also estimatedthat in 2022 about 49,830 people (25,970 men and 23,860 women) will die of pancreaticcancer. [154] Pancreatic cancer accounts for about 3 percent of all cancers in the US and about 7 percent of all cancer deaths. Pancreatic cancer is one of the deadliest cancers. The general five-year survival rate is 11 percent.[155]

The pancreas is a small organ that is located between the lower part of the stomach and the beginning portion of the small intestine. The pancreas has two major functions—the production of digestive enzymes

152 "Key Statistics About Stomach Cancer," American Cancer Society, https://1ref.us/20f (accessed June 6, 2022).

153 J van Beijnum et al., "Insulin-like Growth Factor Axis Targeting In Cancer and Tumour Angiogenesis—The Missing Link," *Biological Reviews* 92 (2017), 1755–1768, https://1ref.us/20g (accessed June 6, 2022).

154 "Pancreatic Risk Factore," American Cancer Society, https://1ref.us/20h (accessed June 6, 2022).

155 "Pancreatic Cancer : Statistics," Cancer.Net, https://1ref.us/20i (accessed June 6, 2022).

and hormones. The most important hormone that the pancreas produces is insulin. Insulin is needed for the regulation of blood sugar levels.

Researchers at Case Western Reserve University School of Medicine in Cleveland, OH, have identified the prion as a biomarker for pancreatic cancer.[156] If prion sounds familiar, it is because prions are the structures that cause Mad Cow Disease. With this latest discovery of the role of prions in pancreatic cancer, it becomes more and more clear that animal flesh and animal products are far more dangerous and involved in diseases than many want to admit. The prion basically hijacks the cells and causes the tumor to grow aggressively.

A recent study published in the Journal of the National Cancer Institute concluded that animal fat in the diet is associated with an increased pancreatic cancer risk. This was not a small study with just a handful of subjects. The study consisted of 525,473 people.[157]

Now we know of three ways in which the pancreas can be attacked as a result of consuming animal products. The first way, as discussed in the section on diabetes, the bovine serum album can attach to the pancreas and cause the pancreas to be recognized as "not self" and be prone to attack by the body. The second way is for prions to get into the pancreatic cells and hijack them, causing aggressive growth of the pancreatic tumors. The third way is the impact that IGF-1 impacts pancreatic cancer cell growth.

Given the role of animals that milk and animal products play in pancreatic cancer, is it really worth the risk of consuming them?

Ovarian Cancer

Ovarian cancer is the fifth leading cause of cancer-related deaths in women ages thirty-five toseventy-four. An estimated one woman in seventy-eight will develop ovarian cancer during herlifetime. The American Cancer Society estimates that in 2022 there will be over 19,880 new cases of ovarian cancer diagnosed this year and that more than 12,810 women will die from ovariancancer this year. This cancer mainly develops in older

---

156 "Prion Protein Identified As Novel Early Pancreatic Cancer Biomarker," Case Western Reserve University, ScienceDaily, 18 August 2009, https://1ref.us/20j (accessed June 6, 2022).
157 "Dietary Fat Linked to Pancreatic Cancer," *Journal of the National Cancer Institute*, June 27, 2009, Science Daily, https://1ref.us/20k (accessed June 6, 2022).

women. About half of the women who arediagnosed with ovarian cancer are sixty-three years or older. It is more common in white womenthan African American women.[158]

When a woman is diagnosed and treated in the earliest stages of this disease, the five-year survival rate is over 90 percent. Due to ovarian cancer's non-specific symptoms and lack of early detection tests, about 20 percent of all cases are found early, meaning in stage I or II. If caught in stage III or higher, the survival rate can be as low as 28 percent. Due to the nature of the disease, each woman diagnosed with ovarian cancer has a different profile, and it is impossible to provide a general prognosis.[159] Ovarian cancer is cancer that forms in the tissues of the ovaries, the female reproductive organs that contain eggs. There are two basic forms of ovarian cancer. The ovarian epithelial carcinoma begins in the cells on the surface of the ovary. The malignant germ cell tumor begins in the egg cells. There are more than 20,000 new cases of ovarian cancer and more than 14,000 deaths from ovarian cancer each year.

A study conducted in Sweden and one conducted among African American women showed that consuming lactose and dairy products was positively linked to ovarian cancer.[160][161] The Iowa Women's Health Study found that women who consumed more than one glass of milk per day had a 73 percent greater chance of developing ovarian cancer than women who drank less than one glass per day.[162] A large study published in the British Journal of Cancer identified 22,788 people who were lactose intolerant and found that those who avoided dairy because they were lactose intolerant had a lower incidence of lung, breast, and ovarian cancers than their family members who did not avoid dairy. The researchers suggest that avoiding

158 "Key Statistics for Ovarian Cancer," American Cancer Society, https://1ref.us/20l (accessed June 6, 2022).

159 "What Is Ovarian Cancer?" National Ovarian Cancer Coalition, https://1ref.us/20m (accessed June 6, 2022).

160 S Larsson, L Bergkvist, A Wolk, "Milk and Lactose Intakes and Ovarian Cancer Risk In the Swedish Mammography Cohort," *The American Journal of Clinical Nutrition* 80, no. 5 (November 2004): 1353–1357, https://1ref.us/20n (accessed June 6, 2022).

161 B Qin et al, "Dairy, Calcium, Vitamin D and Ovarian Cancer Risk In African -American Women," *British Journal of Cancer* 115, no. 9 (October 2016): 1122–1130, https://1ref.us/20o (accessed June 6, 2022).

162 L Kushi et al., "Prospective Study of Diet and Ovarian Cancer," *American Journal of Epidemiology* 149, no. 1 (January 1999): 12–31,

the saturated fat and extra hormones found in dairy products is protective against certain types of cancer.[163]

One culprit in milk that plays a role in ovarian cancer is the sugar galactose. Lactose, the sugar found in milk, is a disaccharide because it is composed of two sugars, glucose and galactose. Galactose has been linked to ovarian cancer since it appears to be toxic to ovarian cells.[164] Galactose is also linked to infertility. However, the real culprit appears to be the saturated fat that is in milk and not the sugar galactose.[165]

When it comes to milk period and not just various components of milk, a study found that women who consumed four or more servings of total dairy products a day had a risk of serous ovarian cancer twice that of women who consumed fewer than two servings of total dairy products per day.[166]

In a study out of Sweden, a total of 22,788 individuals with lactose intolerance were identified. In this large cohort study, people with lactose intolerance, characterized by low consumption of milk and other dairy products, had decreased risks of lung, breast, and ovarian cancers.[167]

Research involving the data from the Harvard Nurse Study has implicated galactose as a factor in ovarian cancer. Lactose, milk sugar, is composed of two sugars, galactose and glucose. Whole milk is lower in milk sugar than skim and lowfat milk.

Prostate Cancer

When I think about prostate cancer, it is easy for tears to well up within my eyes. My best friend, who also played the role of grandfather, uncle, confidant, father, advisor, and mentor, passed away as a result of prostate cancer. He was one of the rarest types of men who ever walked upon the

163 J Ji, J Sundquist, K Sundquist, "Lactose Intolerance and Risk of Lung, Breast and Ovarian Cancers: Aetiological Clues from a Population-Based Study In Sweden," *British Journal of Cancer* 112, no. 1 (January 2015): 149–152, https://1ref.us/20p (accessed June 6, 2022).

164 D Cramer et al., "A Case-control Study of Galactose Consumption and Metabolism In Relation to Ovarian Cancer," *Cancer Epidemiology, Biomarkers and Prevention* 9, no. 1 (January 2000): 95–101, https://1ref.us/20q (accessed June 6, 2022).

165 P Webb et al., "Milk Consumption, Galactose Metabolism and Ovarian Cancer (Australia)," *CCC* 9, no. 6 (December 1998): 637–644, https://1ref.us/20r (accessed June 6, 2022).

166 Larsson, "Milk and Lactose Intakes."

167 Ji, "Lactose Intolerance."

face of the earth. I watched as the disease progressed from his diagnosis until his demise. It was gut-wrenching to watch a healthy man slowly deteriorate to the point he was no longer able to stand or walk on his own. One of my favorite uncles also passed away from prostate cancer. Like my best friend, my uncle Vernon was a strong, healthy man and slowly deteriorated to the point of being bedridden and unaware of his surroundings.

The prostate is a small gland, about the size of a walnut, that is located just under the bladder and in front of the rectum. The prostate produces fluid that makes up the bulk of seminal plasma. As the prostate enlarges, it begins to press against the urethra (the tube in the penis from which urine flows), thereby impeding the flow of urine. This is what is generally responsible for the dribbling and frequent urination that older men often experience.

Research is showing that the prostate cancer that afflicts blacks is different than that which afflicts whites. It is also located in a different area of the prostate and tends to be more malignant. The problem then becomes one of screening. The generic screening that has been in place may very well miss the cancer blacks have.

Prostate cancer is the second most common cancer among men. It is second only to skin cancer. The American Cancer Society's estimates for prostate cancer in the United States for 2020 that there would be about 191,930 new cases of prostate cancer and about 33,330 deaths from prostate cancer. Currently, there are more than 3.1 million men living in the United States who have been diagnosed with prostate cancer. Approximately one man in nine will be diagnosed with prostate cancer during his lifetime. Prostate cancer is more likely to develop in older men and in African-American men. About 60 percent of the cases are diagnosed in men who are sixty-five or older, and it is rare in men under forty. The average age at diagnosis is about sixty-six. Prostate cancer is the second leading cause of cancer death in American men, second only to lung cancer. It is estimated that one man in forty-one will die of prostate cancer.[168] In a recent study in the *American Journal of Clinical Nutrition,* it was determined that high intakes of dairy products increase the risk for prostate cancer. Researchers analyzed data from thirty-two

168 "Key Statistics for Prostate Cancer," American Cancer Society, https://1ref.us/20s (accessed June 6, 2022).

different studies and found total dairy products, total milk, low-fat milk, cheese, and dietary calcium intakes were incrementally associated with an increased risk for prostate cancer.[169] In data from The Physicians Health Study, 21,660 participants were tracked for 28 years, and the data revealed an increased risk of prostate cancer for those who consumed 2.5 or more servings of dairy products per day, compared with those who consumed less than 0.5 servings a day.[170]

Researchers from Harvard Medical School and the University of California completed a major study aimed at determining if IGF-1 and IGFBP-3 levels can predict the risk of developing advanced-stage prostate cancer. Their study involved 530 patients with prostate cancer and 534 controls matched for sex and smoking status. All participants were part of the Physicians' Health Study and were between the ages of forty and eighty-four years at enrollment in 1982. Nearly 15,000 of the men provided blood samples that were stored for future analysis. By the end of 1995, 786 cases of prostate cancer had been diagnosed among the 14,916 participants (5.2%). Sufficient blood plasma for IGF-1 and IGFBP-3 analysis was available for 530 of the cases and their matched 534 controls. The diagnosis of prostate cancer was made an average of nine years after the drawing of the blood samples.[171]

There has not been much research regarding post-diagnostic dairy intake and prostate cancer survival. One of the key players in prostate cancer is estrogen. Fat has a role in the amount of estrogen in the body.[172, 173] Milk is high in saturated fat, and its consumption is significantly associated with surviving prostate cancer. When comparing the consumption of saturated

---

169 D Aune, D Rosenblatt, D Chan, A Vieira, R Vieira, D Greenwood, L Vatten, T Norat, "Dairy Products, Calcium, and Prostate Cancer Risk: A Systematic Review and Meta-analysis of Cohort Studies," *The Journal of American Clinical Nutrition* 101, no. 1 (January 2015): 87–117, https://1ref.us/20t (accessed June 6, 2022).

170 Y Song et al., "Whole Milk Intake Associated with Prostate Cancer-specific Mortality among U.S. Male Physicians," *The Journal of Nutrition* 143, no. 2 (February 2013): 189–196, https://1ref.us/20u (accessed June 6, 2022).

171 J Chan et al., "Insulin-like Growth Factor-I (IGF-I) and IGF Binding Protein-3 as Predictors of Advanced-stage Prostate Cancer," *Journal of the National Cancer Institute* 94, no. 14 (July 2002): 1099–1106, https://1ref.us/20v (accessed June 6, 2022).

172 P Hill, E Wynder, H Garnes, A Walker, "Environmental Factors, Hormone Status, and Prostatic Cancer," *Prventive Medicine* 9, no. 5 (September 1980): 657–666, https://1ref.us/20w (accessed June 6, 2022).

173 E Hamalainen, P Adlercerutaz, P Puska, P Pietinen, "Diet and Serum Hormones in Healthy Men," *Journal of Steroid Beiochemistry* 20, no. 1 (January 1984): 459–464, https://1ref.us/20x (accessed June 6, 2022).

fat in men, it was discovered that men in the upper tercile of saturated fat consumption had three times the risk of dying from prostate cancer than those in the lower tercile. The findings of the study above suggest that, if saturated fat is causally related to disease-specific survival, something as simple as a moderate reduction in saturated fat intake below 10 percent of energy should reduce the risk of dying from prostate cancer.[174] One study evaluated intake of total, high-fat, and low-fat dairy after prostate cancer diagnosis in relation to disease-specific and total mortality. The study included 926 men from the Physicians' Health Study diagnosed with non-metastatic prostate cancer between 1982 and 2000 who completed a diet questionnaire a median of five years after diagnosis and were followed thereafter for a median of ten years to assess mortality. During the time of the study of 8,903 person-years of follow-up, 333 men died, fifty-six due to prostate cancer. The research yielded an astonishing result, men who consumed three or more servings per day of total dairy products had a 76 percent higher risk of total mortality and a 141 percent higher risk of prostate cancer-specific mortality compared to men who consumed less than one dairy product per day.[175]

> Milk is high in saturated fat, and its consumption is significantly associated with surviving prostate cancer.

Data from a study of 14,916 male physicians showed that men with the highest levels of IGF-1 had more than four times the risk of prostate cancer than those with the lowest levels. The researchers noted a strong association between IGF-1 and IGFBP-3 levels and the risk of advanced prostate cancer. However, the researchers did not find such an association with early-stage disease. The research showed that men with IGF levels in the highest quartile had a 5.1 times higher risk of later developing advanced stage prostate cancer than did men in the lowest quartile. Men with IGFBP-3 levels in the highest quartile had a five times lower risk of later advanced stage cancer. Advanced stage prostate cancer was defined as stage C (extraprostatic, but no evidence of distant metastases) or stage D (distant metastatic or fatal). Approximately 10 percent of the total 530

---

174 Y Fradet et al., "Dietary Fat and Prostate Cancer Progresion and Survival," *European Urology* 35, no. 5–6 (1999): 388–391, https://1ref.us/20y (accessed June 6, 2022).

175 M Yang et al., "Dairy Intake After Prostate Cancer Diagnosis In Relation to Disease-specific and Total Mortality," *International Journal of Cancer* 137, no. 10 (November 2015): 2462–2469, https://1ref.us/20z (accessed June 6, 2022).

cases were stage D. The research seems to point to the possibility that IGF-1 not only stimulates tumor initiation and growth but may also facilitate invasion and metastases. The researchers conclude that measurement of IGF-1 and IGFBP-3 levels may predict the risk of advanced stage prostate cancer years before the cancer is actually diagnosed and may thus be helpful in aiding decision making about treatment.[176]

It should not come as a surprise that since milk is generally from pregnant cows, it contains large amounts of estrogen.[177] The particular estrogen found in milk that is at issue is 17 -estradiol. This estrogen works as a carcinogen for prostate cancer. Another chemical of concern that is in high levels in cow's milk is cow's milk is insulin-like growth factor (IGF)-I because it too plays a role in prostate cancer risk due to its role in the growth of cancer cells. In a human study, plasma IGF-I concentration increased by 10 percent when healthy subjects consumed cow's milk.[178]

Studies show that populations that consume the greatest amount of animal protein, including whole milk dairy products, also experience the highest rates of prostate cancer death. A recent study in the British Journal of Cancer showed that a mere 35-gram increase in the consumption of dairy protein was associated with an astounding 32 percent increase in the risk of prostate cancer.[179] Calcium from dairy products was also positively associated with risk, but not calcium from other food sources. In addition to increased amounts of animal protein and calcium. Evidence from studies of Chinese men living in both China and North America show that saturated fat and animal fat consumption are linked to increased prostate cancer risk.[180, 181]

176 W Cromie, "Growth Factor Raises Cancer Risk," *The Harvard Gazette*, April 22, 1999, https://1ref.us/210 (accessed June 6, 2022).

177 R Heap, M Hamon, "Oestrone Sulphate In Milk as an Indicator of a Viable Conceptus In Cows," *The British Veterinary Journal* 135, no. 4 (July/August 1979): 355–363, https://1ref.us/211 (accessed June 6, 2022).

178 R Heaney et al., "Dietary Changes Favorably Affect Bone Remodeling In Older Adults," *Journal of the American Dietetic Association* 99, no. 10 (October 1999): 1228–1233, https://1ref.us/212 (accessed June 6, 2022).

179 A Whittemore et al., "Prostate Cancer In Relation to Diet, Physical Activity, and Body Size In Blacks, Whites, and Asians In the United States and Canada," *JNCI* 87, no. 9 (May 1995): 652–661, https://1ref.us/213 (accessed June 6, 2022).

180 M Lee et al., "Case-control Study of Diet and Prostate Cancer In China," *CCC* 9, no. 6 (December 1998): 545–552, https://1ref.us/214 (accessed June 6, 2022).

181 N Allen et al., "Animal Foods, Protein, Calcium and Prostate Cancer Risk: The European Prospective Investigation Into Cancer and Nutrition," *British Journal of Cancer* 98, no. 9 (May 2008): 1574–1581, https://1ref.us/215 (accessed June 6, 2022).

Lung Cancer

Lung cancer is divided into two main groups, small cell lung cancer (SCLC), the less common, and non-small cell lung cancer (NSCLC). About 13 percent of all lung cancers are SCLC, and 84 percent are NSCLC. Lung cancer is the second most common cancer in both men and women, aside from skin cancer. In men, lung cancer is second only to prostate cancer, while in women, breast cancer is more common. The American Cancer Society's estimates for lung cancer in the United States for 2022 there will be: 236,740 new cases of lung cancer (117,910 in men and 118,830 in women) and approximately 130,180 deaths from lung cancer (68,820 in men and 61,360 in women).[182]

Lung cancer is a disease that mainly occurs in older people, those sixty-five and older. Lung cancer is rarely diagnosed among people younger than forty-five. The average age of people when diagnosed is about seventy. Lung cancer is by far the leading cause of cancer death among both men and women, making up almost 25 percent of all cancer deaths. Each year, more people die of lung cancer than of <u>colon</u>, breast, and prostate cancers combined.[183]

Overall, the chance that a man will develop lung cancer in his lifetime is about one in fifteen; for a woman, the risk is about one in seventeen. For smokers the risk is much higher, while for non-smokers, the risk is lower. Black men are about 12 percent more likely to develop lung cancer than white men. The rate is about 16 percent lower in black women than in white women. Black and white women have lower rates than men, but the gap is closing. The lung cancer rate has been dropping among men over the past few decades, but only for about the last decade in women. Despite their overall risk of lung cancer being higher, black men are less likely to develop SCLC than are white men.[184]

The fact that the consumption of milk has been associated with lung cancer came even as a shock to me! We know that smoking causes cancer, but why is it that American men over the age of fifty have much higher rates of lung cancer than Japanese men of the same age?

---

182 "Lung Cancer Survival Rates," American Cancer Society, https://1ref.us/216 (accessed June 6, 2022).
183 "Lung Cancer Survival Rates."
184 "Lung Cancer Survival Rates."

Given that BLV has been found in human blood, it is only a matter of time before we realize the extent to which BLV is involved in many cancers. Recently, BLV DNA was found in non-small cell lung cancer.[185]

The Japanese provide a cornucopia of research related to diet and cancer because of their historically low consumption of meat and animal products. Japanese men born prior to 1950 consumed virtually no milk. Japanese men born before 1960 drank very little milk. Milk and milk products simply were not a staple of the Japanese diet up to that period of time. Dietary research began in the 1940s. Since that time, every year, thousands upon thousands of Japanese have their diets analyzed. In 1975, 21,707 Japanese were studied. After studying these people, the researchers discovered that the per-capita yearly dietary intake of dairy products in 1950 was just 5.5 pounds. By 1975, the per-capita yearly dietary intake of dairy products had skyrocketed to 117.4 pounds of milk and dairy products per year.

During the 25-year period from 1950 to 1975, the consumption of dairy products increased by a factor of 21. During this period, the rate of lung cancer jumped approximately 250 percent![186] According to researchers, again, IGF-1 has been implicated as a major player in yet another form of cancer—lung cancer.

Non-Hodgkin's Lymphoma

Scientists at Yale University conducted a seven-year study on 1,318 women in Connecticut that determined that the women with diets high in fiber had low rates of lymphatic cancer. Conversely, the women with diets that included high amounts of dairy and animal products had higher rates of lymphatic cancer. Tongzhang Zheng, ScD, head of the division of environmental health sciences at the Yale School of Public Health in New Haven, Connecticut, collected detailed dietary information from 601 Connecticut women with non-Hodgkin's lymphoma and from 717 similar women without cancer.

---

185 L Robinson et al., "Molecular Evidence of Viral DNA In Non-small Cell Lung Cancer and Non-neoplastic Lung," *British Journal of Cancer* 115, no. 4 (August 2016): 497–504, https://1ref.us/217 (accessed June 6, 2022).
186 O Gersten, J Wilmoth, "The Cancer Transition In Japan Since 1951," *Demographic Research* 7, no. 5 (August 2002): 271–306, https://1ref.us/218 (accessed June 6, 2022).

"What we found is if a person has a higher intake of animal protein, they will have a higher risk of non-Hodgkin's lymphoma," Zheng tells Web. "And people who have a higher intake of saturated fat have an increased risk. On the other hand, if you have higher-than-average intake of dietary fiber—particularly if you frequently eat vegetables and fruits with a high fiber content—you have a reduced risk of non-Hodgkin's lymphoma."[187]

---

187 X Han et al., "Vegetable and Fruit Intake and Non-Hodgkin Lymphoma Survival In Connecticut Women," *Leukemia and Lymphoma* 51, no. 6 (June 2010): 1047–1054, https://1ref.us/219 (accessed June 6, 2022).

Chapter 9

DEMENTIA? I FORGOT ...

It is estimated that the brain has approximately 100,000,000,000,000 (one hundred billion) synaptic connections. Each neuron (brain cell) can have a multitude of synapses and thus are able to communicate with hundreds of thousands of other neurons in a matter of microseconds. It's logical then that the more and better connections or synapses and dendrites a nerve cell has, the greater its capacity for transmitting messages and processing information. This translates into increased intelligence and better mental functioning.

Scientists have discovered approximately fifty chemicals in the brain called neurotransmitters. Neurotransmitters are the essence of the individual. They form paths that carry your every thought, inclination, feeling, etc., throughout the vast neuronal network. Neurotransmitters are manufactured in the brain cell. It stands to reason then that there is a solid connection between what the body takes in as food has a profound impact on the type of neurotransmitters the brain cells manufacture. As in any manufacturing process, the end product is dictated by the raw materials available. So, it is with the brain cell. Consider the neurotransmitters serotonin, acetylcholine, and dopamine. Serotonin is known as the "good-mood" neurotransmitter. It increases memory and protects the brain from a phenomenon called excitotoxicity. Its basic building block is tryptophan. Tryptophan is an amino acid found in many foods. Acetylcholine is vital for memory. It relies on choline, a substance found in soybeans, as its basic building block. Dopamine is necessary for motor coordination. Dopamine relies on the substance tyrosine, which is often found in foods high in protein. In addition, there are other chemicals, which act to limit the amount and determine the nature and function of neurotransmitters.

One such chemical is folic acid, a B vitamin. Without the right nutrients in the right amounts, disaster awaits.

The fascinating news is that you can create more connections-synapses, dendrites, and receptors—through diet, supplements, mental exercise, and physical exercise. The bad news is that the brain can be compromised through diet, lack of supplements, and lack of mental and physical exercise.

There are several roads that lead to dementia. However, we will concern ourselves primarily with the dietary aspects of the ingestion of meat and animal products, namely saturated fat, cholesterol, and excess protein. As you will soon see, these are instrumental in causing low-level inflammation, high blood pressure, and cerebral vascular disease, all of which are implicated in the development of dementia.

Alzheimer's has skyrocketed from near obscurity to sixth place as the leading cause of death in the U.S. In 2000, 49,558 people died of Alzheimer's Disease. By 2017, the number of people who died from Alzheimer's more than doubled to 121,404. Currently, there are more than 5.8 million people in the U.S. age sixty-five and up with Alzheimer's. This number is expected to nearly triple to 14 million by the year 2050. Nearly two-thirds of those with Alzheimer's in the U.S. are women. Older African-Americans are about twice as likely to have Alzheimer's or other dementias as older whites. The cost to the country is staggering, with no end in sight. In 20201, dementias cost the U.S. $355 billion. It is estimated that by 2050, the cost will more than triple to $1.1 trillion.[188] There are several factors responsible for this alarming rise in the prevalence of Alzheimer's. One factor is the ingestion of saturated fats and cholesterol. A high intake of saturated fat and cholesterol and a low intake of polyunsaturated fatty acids have been related to an increased risk of cardiovascular disease. Cardiovascular disease has been associated with dementia. Vascular dementia is widely considered the second most common cause of dementia after Alzheimer's disease, accounting for 5 percent to 10 percent of cases.[189]

---

188 "Alzheimer's Disease Facts and Figures," Alzheimer's Association, https://1ref.us/21a (accessed June 6, 2022).
189 "Alzheimer's Disease Facts and Figures."

Fat – Friend and foe?

The brain is 60 percent fat, the fattiest organ in the body! That being the case, the type of fat that is in the diet will have an impact on the brain. A diet high in "good fats" found in nuts and vegetable oils seems to lower the risk of Alzheimer's disease. Eating fried foods and other "bad fats" increase the risk.

With the ingestion of milk comes the ingestion of saturated fats and cholesterol. Data from the Rotterdam Study showed that high intake of total fat, saturated fat, and cholesterol was associated with an increased risk of Alzheimer's. Saturated fat leads to chemical reactions, which result in radicals. These radicals then cause damage to the mitochondria and lining of the blood vessels. In addition, the fat and excess proteins lead to low-level inflammation of blood vessels in the brain. Furthermore, fat eventually causes a decrease in blood flow to areas of the brain. The decrease in blood flow is one of the factors that leads to Alzheimer's.

> Fat eventually causes a decrease in blood flow to areas of the brain. The decrease in blood flow is one of the factors that leads to Alzheimer's.

When the brain gets "bad" fat, the brain changes physically. The outer membrane of the brain cell becomes rigid and often changes in shape. The message-sending parts of the cell known as dendrites are changed physically. It has been demonstrated in laboratory studies that animals fed high amounts of saturated fat have a decline in cognitive function. Furthermore, neurotransmitters are inhibited in their task due to their inability to enter the now rigid brain cells.

The chief "bad" fat is saturated animal fat. Studies demonstrate that laboratory animals that were fed lots of saturated fat in the form of lard do not learn as quickly or perform as well on a multitude of memory tests. Laboratory animals fed polyunsaturated soybean oil did much better on the tests than their saturated fat-fed counterparts. The lard-fed animals had problems with both long-term as well as short-term memory. The studies demonstrate that as the amount of saturated fat is increased in the diet, the severity of brain and hence memory malfunction increases. With animals on a diet that was composed of 10 percent saturated fat, learning was almost non-existent.

A study looked at the association between fat intake and incident dementia among participants, age fifty-five years or older, from the population-based prospective Rotterdam Study. Food intake of 5,386 nondemented participants was assessed at baseline with a semiquantitative food-frequency questionnaire. At baseline and after an average of 2.1 years of follow-up, the participants were screened for dementia with a three-step protocol that included a clinical examination. Dementia with a vascular component was most strongly related to total fat and saturated fat. This study suggests that a high saturated fat and cholesterol intake increases the risk of dementia, whereas fish consumption may decrease this risk.[190]

Saturated fat leads to chemical reactions that result in radicals. These radicals then cause damage to the mitochondria and lining of the blood vessels. In addition, the fat and excess proteins lead to low-level inflammation of blood vessels in the brain. Furthermore, fat eventually causes a decrease in blood flow to areas of the brain. The decrease in blood flow is one of the factors that leads to Alzheimer's.

With respect to human studies and not laboratory animal studies, researchers at Rush-Presbyterian St. Luke's Medical Center in Chicago studied 815 seniors without Alzheimer's. After six years, 131 developed Alzheimer's. It was discovered that those who ate a lot of saturated fats, fats found in meat and dairy, were twice as likely to develop AD than those who ate small amounts.[191] Those who consumed large amounts of polyunsaturated fats, fats found in vegetables and nuts, reduced their risk by 70 percent compared with those who ate small amounts of these fats.

Chronic Low-Level Inflammation

Researchers now implicate chronic low-level inflammation in neurological damage, including Alzheimer's disease. It is no secret that people who take anti-inflammatory drugs have lower rates of Alzheimer's disease. Aspirin, vitamin C and E, and cholesterol-lowering statin drugs work as anti-inflammatory agents. Inflammation also develops from prostaglandins

---

190 S Kalmijn et al., "Dietary Fat Intake and the Risk of Incident Dementia In the Rotterdam Study," *Annals of Neurology* 42, no. 5 (November 1997): 776–782, https://1ref.us/21b (accessed June 6, 2022).

191 J Davis, "Fat In Diet Linked With Alzheimer's," WebMD, https://1ref.us/21c (accessed June 6, 2022); E Manuelidis, L Manuelidis, "Suggested Links Between Different Types of Dementias," *Alzheimer Disease and Associated Disorders* 3, no. 1–2 (Spring/Summer 1989): 100–109, https://1ref.us/21d (accessed June 6, 2022).

from fatty acids. Series 2 prostaglandins are derived from arachidonic acid found in meats and other animal products and lead to the kidneys retaining salt that leads to increased blood pressure and causes inflammation.

When fats are metabolized, numerous byproducts are created. One such group of byproducts are eicosanoids which are prostaglandins, leukotrienes, and cytokines. In addition, multitudinous free radicals are produced. These products initiate inflammation. Some prostaglandins have been named "neurotoxins" because they kill brain cells.

Arachidonic acid, a pro-inflammatory agent produced by the conversion of some fats, also stimulates the production of glutamate. Glutamate has the dual role of being a neurotransmitter as well as a brain cell destroyer. Glutamate in excess causes cells to fire until they die. During this process, free radicals are produced, and the calcium balance in the cell is disturbed and sent to toxic levels leading to cellular death. This process is known as "excitotoxicity." Just about the only thing that can save a cell experiencing excitotoxicity is for it to have the many radicals removed by antioxidant products.

Cerebral Vascular Disease

What are commonly known as "strokes" are more properly referred to as cerebral vascular accidents, or more succinctly, CVAs. This disorder is the direct result of the brain cells not receiving their much-needed supply of oxygen and nutrients. Subsequent to their deprivation of oxygen and nutrients, these cells will die, and unlike other cells in the body, brain cells will not regenerate.

As stated earlier, in atherosclerosis the passageway of the blood vessel becomes narrowed as a result of the atheromas attaching to and accumulating on the wall of the blood vessel. This action changes the normally smooth surface of the wall of the blood vessel to a rough one, thereby making the surface conducive for the formation of blood clots. Once blood clots form, they tend to continue to grow. As platelets become enmeshed in the fibronin threads, the platelets start to disintegrate. This results in the release of more thromboplastin, which, in turn, causes more clotting, which enmeshes more platelets, and so on, resulting in a vicious circle. These clots can continue to grow until they finally block the passageway of the blood vessel completely. Furthermore, these clots can break off and travel freely through the blood vessel until they become lodged on the wall and grow to form another large clot. This is particularly dangerous when it happens in the brain because of the many small blood vessels contained in it, the inability of modern medicine to reach these impaired vessels, and the inability of the brain cells to regenerate.

Atherosclerosis can also play a key role in cerebral vascular accidents when atheromas collect on the wall of blood vessels in the brain and continue to grow. If the growth of these atheromas continues uninterrupted, they will eventually preclude the flow of blood through the vessel completely or to a serious degree. In addition, the atheromas can break off and travel through the blood vessels of the brain freely, as in the case of blood clots, until they become lodged, thereby restricting the flow of blood, resulting in a cerebral vascular accident or stroke.

Cerebral vascular accidents may also be caused by cerebral hemorrhages. Cerebral hemorrhages result when blood vessels in the brain rupture. The consequence of this happening is an interference in blood flow as well as the accumulation of blood in the affected area.

In 1998 158,100 people died as a result of cerebral vascular disease. Approximately 1.7 percent of men and 1.4 percent of women between the ages of forty-five to sixty-four have cerebral vascular disease. For those sixty-five years of age and over, the percent of men increases to 5.6 percent and to 5.8 percent for women. Autopsy reports show that 60-90 percent of Alzheimer's victims also have cerebral vascular disease.

Strokes result in the death of areas in the brain. These dead areas will not regenerate and will be replaced by scar tissue. Depending upon the amount and the area of the brain that was damaged, strokes may leave their victims completely or partially paralyzed. An individual suffering from a stroke may also experience a condition known as hemianopsia, the ability to see only half of their normal visual field.

Homocysteine

As mentioned earlier, homocysteine is an amino acid that is formed in the liver after ingesting another amino acid called methionine. Animal protein has two to three times the amount of methionine as plant protein. Consequently, those who consume animal products are much more likely to have increased levels of homocysteine, which leads to a condition known as hyperhomocysteinemia. Hyperhomocysteinemia. is of concern because it is associated with Alzheimer's disease due to cerebral vascular disease.

High Blood Pressure (Hypertension)

Hypertension is instrumental in reducing the size of the brain as well as causing damage to the brain. This results in mental decline often associated with aging.

Oxidative Stress

Alzheimer's disease is preceded by a prodromal phase characterized by mild cognitive impairment. Individuals with mild cognitive impairment have increased brain oxidative damage before the onset of symptomatic dementia.

Oxidative stress leads to the accumulation of free radicals, which leads to excessive lipid (fat) peroxidation and neuronal degeneration in certain parts of the brain. In addition, the accumulation of free radicals damage DNA, the proteins, and lipid membranes. The aggregation of beta-amyloid is increased by oxidative stress. Oxidative stress is instrumental in the conversion of soluble to insoluble beta-amyloids.

Insulin Resistance

Studies have shown that people who eat lots of saturated fats are likely to develop insulin resistance, a situation in which the cells are unable to utilize glucose effectively. Insulin resistance is also a condition that precedes diabetes. It is, in effect, a pre-diabetic state. This condition is responsible for the cells not being able to utilize glucose effectively, and as a consequence, cells throughout the body begin to starve. This leads to a host of symptoms related to blood sugar imbalance. Saturated fats impair insulin sensitivity. Decreasing saturated fatty acids and increasing monounsaturated fatty acids improves insulin sensitivity.

Multi-Infarct Dementia

Multi-infarct dementia (MID) makes up about 15 percent of the cases of dementia and is often, no pun intended, confused with Alzheimer's and delirium as result of its unpredictable clinical course. MID results from the interruption of the supply of blood to the brain, usually due to cardiovascular disease, cerebrovascular disease, and hypertension. Once deprived of oxygen and nutrients, brain cells die quickly. The area of damage is known as an infarct. When a person suffers from numerous infarcts, which result from mini-strokes, MID is the result.

The early signs of MID are headaches, dizziness, and a decline in mental and physical vigor. It has an abrupt onset. In many cases the sufferer will experience sudden confusion followed by gradual "spotty" memory loss. In addition, depending on the part of the brain that is affected, the person with MID may hallucinate and show difficulty with speech and may have seizures. In the later stages of MID, the course of the disease is similar to Alzheimer's and often difficult to distinguish from Alzheimer's.

MID differs from Alzheimer's in that a person suffering from Alzheimer's will have a progressive downward course. Those suffering from MID will have an uneven course. This is because some form of recovery and a plateau often follows each infarct. This disease often develops between the ages of fifty to seventy and is found more often in men than women.

Data from the Nun Study shows that those with brain infarcts had poorer cognitive function and a higher prevalence than those without infarct. Participants with lacunar infarcts in the basal ganglia, thalamus, or deep white matter of the brain had an even higher prevalence of dementia compared to those without infarcts. In addition, the study noted that among all participants, atherosclerosis of the circle of Willis (a major blood vessel in the brain) was strongly associated with lacunar and large brain infarcts.

Alzheimer's Disease in concert with vCJD

If, in fact, Alzheimer's is a disease that afflicts only old people, why is it that the number of people dying from it is disproportionate to the number of aged people in the U.S.? The question uppermost on my mind is what is responsible for such a dramatic increase in the number of cases of people dying from Alzheimer's. Are people who are dying from Alzheimer's really dying from other diseases that are manifested by symptoms that are similar to those of Alzheimer's?

The Centers for Disease Control would have us believe that the alarming increase in the number of deaths from Alzheimer's is due to improved awareness and diagnosis. They are not being open about the possibility that a number of the cases could be something other than Alzheimer's.

The diagnosis of Alzheimer's disease is complicated by the likelihood of it being misdiagnosed, even by neurologists. Two neurologists independently reviewed the clinical records of fifty-four demented patients autopsied at the University of Pittsburgh. They did not have knowledge of the patient's identity, clinical, or pathological diagnoses. Both clinicians were correct in 63 percent of the cases, only one was correct in 17 percent, and in 20 percent of the cases, neither was correct. These results show that patients with a clinical diagnosis of dementia, the cause or origin cannot be predicted during life. Alzheimer's disease can only be definitely diagnosed upon death when the brain can be examined microscopically to view changes characteristic of the disease. A lead researcher in finding a viral component to Mad Cow disease, Laura Manuelidis, noted as early as 1989, "In our own neuropathological material, in 46 cases diagnosed clinically as AD (Alzheimer's disease), 6 cases were proven to be CJD at autopsy." In another post-mortem study, three out of twelve "Alzheimer" patients actually died from a spongiform encephalopathy.[192]

Given the foregoing, it is clear that what was often diagnosed as Alzheimer's disease was actually something else in a considerable percentage of cases ranging from 13 percent to 37 percent. If we hold to those percentages, it will mean that of the 72,432 deaths from Alzheimer's disease in 2006, 9,416 to 26,800 were the result of an Alzheimer's-like disease. More frightening is that of the 15,000,000 cases of Alzheimer's cases that are estimated to exist in the U.S. in the year 2050, anywhere from 2,000,000 to 5,500,000 will not be Alzheimer's but something equally deleterious to the brain and perhaps even more potent in that it will attack people at a younger age.

It is generally agreed by experts that Alzheimer's begins with the accumulation of amyloid beta protein. Amyloid beta protein results from a larger protein called amyloid precursor protein (APP). APP is a normal protein found in the membrane of neurons. Enzymes called beta and gamma secretase come along and cut the APP in such a way that the resulting helical fragment, amyloid beta protein, is insoluble rather than soluble.

---

192 F Boller, O Lopez, J Moossy, "Diagnosis of Dementia: Clinicopathologic Correlations," *Neurology* 39, no. 1 (January 1989): 76–79, https://1ref.us/21e (accessed June 6, 2022).

Problems begin as these A-beta fragments begin to bind to one another and accumulate. This occurs when A-beta fragments lose their helical shape and become somewhat flat in structure, stack up, and bind together to form fibrils. The resulting fibrils then bind together to form even larger structures. A-beta fibrils also bind with other proteins like SAP, making a mass that is even less soluble. These masses combine with one another and form plaques. However, new research is showing that in cases of a variant form of Creutzfeldt-Jacob disease (CJD), it, too, has an abnormal neuronal membrane protein, namely, PrPCJD, that produces amyloid plaques. Moreover, to complicate things further, the brain of one with Alzheimer's can become spongy, as with cases of CJD. In other words, there may very well be more people walking around with CJD, Alzheimer's, or both!

As the plaques continue to grow in size and number, they begin to displace brain tissue that leads to the inability to produce the neurotransmitter acetylcholine. Acetylcholine is involved in memory formation. As the amount of acetylcholine in the brain decreases, the brain becomes less able to exchange signals and messages. This leads to a decrease in memory, perception, and the ability to think. At the same time, plaque causes another neurotransmitter, glutamate, to increase in the brain. Glutamate is involved in memory but becomes toxic to neurons when it is in abnormally high levels. Moreover, the remaining brain tissue becomes insensitive to glutamate in the formation of new memories.

A nightmare is slowly unfolding and will be unfolding publicly soon because the numbers involved will be chilling and can no longer be hidden. The nightmare that I am in reference to is the reemergence of foodborne Mycobacterium bovis (bovine tuberculosis) as a vector for Creutzfeldt-Jakob disease, which is the human form of Mad Cow disease. The CDC reported an outbreak of CJD linked to the consumption of meat contaminated "with the agent causing" bovine spongiform encephalopathy (BSE) in a New Jersey racetrack between 1995-2004. Therefore, it is highly likely that a similar pathogenesis for Alzheimer's, CJD, and other spongiform encephalopathies such as Mad Cow disease. This is given credence by the fact that CJD and Alzheimer's often coexist and are thought to differ only by time-dependent physical changes. The fact that Alzheimer's and CJD coexist is not a novel discovery.

Bovine tuberculosis is an umbrella term that includes Mycobacterium bovis and Mycobacterium paratuberculosis, which historically has been the greatest threat to the cattle industry. It is estimated that up to and possibly more than 40 percent of all U.S. dairy herds are infected with paratuberculosis alone. The risk to human health from milk tainted with

> *CJD and Alzheimer's often coexist and are thought to differ only by time-dependent physical changes.*

tuberculosis is not a new phenomenon. The risk has been known for many decades. In fact, it was not too long ago that "tuberlin-tested" was printed on every milk container. In the early 1900s, 25 percent of the adults who died from tuberculosis died from Mycobacterium bovis.

Many investigators linked BSE in cattle with M. bovis and paratuberculosis in clinical, pathologic, and epidemiological studies. Just prior to the Mad Cow outbreak in the United Kingdom, there was an exponential rise in the number of cases of bovine tuberculosis. This leads us to the inescapable conclusion that Alzheimer's, CJD, and Mad Cow are caused by consuming meat and dairy products.

Other types of dementias

Creutzfeldt Jacob Disease (CJD)
CJD is brain disorder that usually occurs due to deposits of infectious proteins called prions. Creutzfeldt-Jakob disease usually has no known cause but can be inherited. It may also be caused by exposure to diseased brain or nervous system tissue, even from such a cornea transplant. Signs and symptoms of this fatal condition usually appear after age sixty. The vCJD has occurred in children as young as fifteen.

Lewy Body Dementia
Lewy bodies are abnormal balloon-like clumps of protein that have been found in the brains of people with Alzheimer's disease and Parkinson's disease. This is one of the more common types of progressive dementia. Common signs and symptoms include acting out one's dreams in sleep, seeing things that aren't there (visual hallucinations), and problems with focus and attention. Other signs include uncoordinated or slow movement, tremors, and rigidity (parkinsonism). The brain changes involve a protein called alpha-synuclein.

Huntington's Disease

Huntington's Disease is characterized by specific types of uncontrolled movements but also includes dementia. Caused by a genetic mutation, this disease causes certain nerve cells in the brain and spinal cord to atrophy. Signs and symptoms, including a severe decline in thinking (cognitive) skills, usually appear as early as around age thirty.

Normal Pressure Hydrocephalus

Normal pressure hydrocephalus (NPH) is an abnormal buildup of cerebrospinal fluid (CSF) in the brain's ventricles or cavities. It occurs if the normal flow of CSF throughout the brain and spinal cord is blocked in some way. This causes the ventricles to enlarge, putting pressure on the brain.

Parkinson's Disease Dementia

Parkinson's Disease is a neurodegenerative condition linked to abnormal structures in the brain. The brain changes involve a protein called alpha-synuclein.

Vascular Dementia

This second most common type of dementia is caused by damage to the vessels that supply blood to your brain. Blood vessel problems can cause strokes or damage the brain in other ways, such as by damaging the fibers in the white matter of the brain. The most common symptoms of vascular dementia include difficulties with problem-solving, slowed thinking, focus, and organization. These tend to be more noticeable than memory loss.

Korsakoff Syndrome

Korsakoff Syndrome is a chronic memory disorder caused by severe deficiency of thiamine (vitamin B-1) and is often associated with the consumption of inordinate amounts of alcohol.

The following disorders lead to symptoms of dementia:

Posterior cortical atrophy resembles changes seen in Alzheimer's disease but in a different part of the brain.

Frontotemporal Dementia is also known as Pick's disease. This is a group of diseases characterized by the breakdown of nerve cells and their connections in the frontal and temporal lobes of the brain, the areas generally associated with personality, behavior, and language. Common symptoms affect behavior, personality, thinking, judgment, language, and movement.

Mixed dementia. Autopsy studies of the brains of people eighty and older who had dementia indicate that many had a combination of several causes, such as Alzheimer's disease, vascular dementia, and Lewy body dementia. Studies are ongoing to determine how having mixed dementia affects symptoms and treatments.

Down Syndrome increases the likelihood of young-onset Alzheimer's.

Normal pressure hydrocephalus occurs when excess cerebrospinal fluid accumulates in the brain.

Chapter 10

BREASTFED, THE BEST FED!

The milk of every species that produces milk that its "baby" or "babies" need to survive has a unique composition designed specifically for its offspring as they develop. The composition of milk changes as the offspring grows and develops.

The dairy industry, from its inception, has tried to fool us into thinking that the milk from a 1,000-pound cow is superior to the human breast milk for feeding babies. Scientists, in their arrogance, think that by taking cow's milk and subjecting it to homogenization, pasteurization, reformulation, and fortification, that somehow this concoction will meet the nutritional needs of growing babies. They are wrong, and one need only look at and consider the misery such garbage placed in the human system has caused. As I've outlined in this book, cow's milk is not suited for human consumption!

Believe it or not, scientists do not know everything, no matter how many initials are behind their name and no matter how much "Ivy" was in the school from which they received their education. If they were so smart, why are they so bent on trying to make something that is so unnatural, natural? The answer is simply pure economics. The dairy industry has made prostitutes out of science and scientists solely for the purpose of making money. Dairy farmers spend tons of money to make tons of milk that is effectively worthless. The value of milk comes only from dumbing down an ignorant and trusting public via "science" into the belief that milk will provide the nutrients that humans need.

There is far more to breastfeeding a baby than science can EVER expect to know, let alone duplicate. There are substances in breast milk that vary in concentration with the growing needs of the baby. Moreover, there are substances in breast milk that scientists have yet to discover, let alone their function. For instance, recently, British scientists discovered that a hormone manufactured in the human breast called pancreatice secretory trypsin inhibitor (PSTI) may be instrumental in protecting and repairing the intestinal mucosa of newborns. There is so much more to learn! However, the simple truth that cannot be escaped is that breastfed babies are the best-fed babies!!!

Having read this far in this book, you can see that the use of cow's milk for human consumption is wasteful, expensive, CRAZY, and DEADLY! Below you will find a multitude of benefits derived from breastfeeding your child rather than formula feeding. I do understand that not all mothers can breastfeed their children. That is not the issue here. The issue is that breastfeeding a child is the best way of feeding it.

Breastfeeding is highly recommended!

It is safe to say that the majority of health professionals and health authorities recommend breastfeeding the newborn for at least six months. Many will go on to say that breastfeeding should go on for a year or more with a gradual introduction of different foods into the baby's diet.[193][194]

Breast milk contains all of the nutrients a baby needs and in the right amount for a baby, not a calf!

What is fascinating is that the mother's breast milk changes over time in harmony with the growth and development of the baby.[195][196]

Breast milk provides an immunity stockpile of antibodies!

Breastfeeding increases mother's risk of breast cancer. Breast milk contains numerous antibodies that help the child in its fight against illness due to bacteria and viruses. The initial composition of breast milk

---

193 "Breastfeeding and the Use of Human Milk," *Pediatrics* 129, no. 3 (March 2012): e827–841, https://1ref.us/21f (accessed June 6, 2022).

194 See A.A.P. Breastfeeding Policy Statement: Breastfeeding and the Use of Human Milk—RE9729, https://1ref.us/21g (accessed June 6, 2022).

195 O Ballard, A Morrow, "Human Milk Composition: Nutrients and Bioactive Factors," *Pediatric Clinics of North America* 60, no. 1 (February 2013): 49–74,

196 L Read et al., "Changes In the Growth-promoting Activity of Human Milk During Lactation," *Pediatric Research* 28, no. 2 (February 1984): 133–139, https://1ref.us/21i (accessed June 6, 2022).

is colostrum. Colostrum is filled with large amounts of antibodies, in particular immunoglobulin A (IgA).[197][198] The protection that the mother gives her child by breastfeeding is not given to children who are fed formula. Studies show that formula-fed babies are more prone to a host of health issues ranging from diarrhea to pneumonia.[199][200][201] For infants, not being breastfed is associated with an increased incidence of infectious morbidity, as well as elevated risks of childhood obesity, type 1 and type 2 diabetes, and leukemia.[202] One of the more common infections babies have is that of ear infections. When a baby is breastfed for three months, there is a reduction of middle ear infections by up to 50 percent.[203] When a baby is breastfed for more than four months, there is a reduction of the risk of hospitalizations for respiratory infections by up to 72 percent.[204] [205]With respect to colds and throat infections, babies breastfed for six months may have a 63percent decrease in risk of getting these infections.[206] [207] When a baby is exclusively breastfed for three to four months, there is a 27 to 42percent decreased risk of asthma, atopic, dermatitis, and eczema.[208] This should come as no surprise because the proteins that the mother is

---

197 W Hurley, P Theil, "Perspectives on Immunoglobulins In Colostrum and Milk," *Nutrients* 3, no. 4 (April 2011): 442–474, https://1ref.us/21j (accessed June 6, 2022).

198 K Sadeharju et al., "Maternal Antibodies In Breast Milk Protect the Child from Enterovirus Infections," *Pediatrics* 119, no. 5 (May 2007): 941–946, https://1ref.us/21k (accessed June 6, 2022).

199 A Stuebe, "The Risks of Not Breastfeeding for Mothers and Infants," *Reviews In Obstetrics and Gynecology* 2, no. 4 (Fall 2009): 222–231, https://1ref.us/21l (accessed June 6, 2022).

200 S Hengstermann et al., "Formula Feeding Is Associated with Increased Hospital Admissions," *Journal of Human Lactation* 26, no. 1 (February 2010): 19–25, https://1ref.us/21m (accessed June 6, 2022).

201 S Huffman, C Combest, "Role of Breast-feeding In the Prevention and Treatment of Diarrhoea," *Journal of Diarrhoeal Diseases Research* 8, no. 3 (September 1990): 68–81, https://1ref.us/21n (accessed June 6, 2022).

202 Stuebe, "The Risks of Not Breastfeeding."

203 L Duijts et al., "Prolonged and Exclusive Breastfeeding Reduces the Risk of Infectious Diseases In Infancy," *Pediatrics* 126, no. 1 (July 2010): e18–25, https://1ref.us/21o (accessed June 6, 2022).

204 S Ip et al., "Breastfeeding and Maternal and Infant Health Outcomes In Developed Countries," *Evidence Report/Technology Assessment* 153 (April 2007): 1–186, https://1ref.us/21t (accessed June 8, 2022).

205 S Ip et al., "A Summary of the Agency for Healthcare Research and Quality's Evidence Report on Breastfeeding In Developed Countries," *Breastfeeding Medicine* (October 2009): s17–30, https://1ref.us/21u (accessed June 7, 2022).

206 Duijts, "Prolonged and Exclusive Breastfeeding."

207 Duijts, "Prolonged and Exclusive Breastfeeding."

208 Ip, "Breastfeeding and Maternal Health."

passing in her milk is unlike those passed by a cow to her calf. The bovine serum albumin present in cow's milk has been associated with diabetes in children. Perhaps that is one reason why babies who are breastfed for at least three months have a decreased risk of contracting type 1 diabetes by up to 30 percent and type 2 diabetes by up 40 percent.[209][210][211]

Formula Feeding is associated with lower I.Q.

We have not begun to scratch the surface regarding the many factors involved in breastfeeding. Studies now are showing that children who are breastfed have higher I.Q.s. A study to support this statement was done in New Zealand. Here an eighteen-year longitudinal study of over 1,000 children found that those who were breastfed as infants had both better intelligence and greater academic achievement than children who were infant-formula fed.[212] The difference in IQ may also be the result of a difference in the way the brain develops in a child that is breastfed, whether it be due to the security and closeness of being with the mother or the nutrients in the breastmilk, or a combination.[213][214][215][216] Studies now are showing that breastfeeding has positive effects on long-term brain development. Such development may lead to fewer behavioral and learning problems as the child grows older.[217]

---

209 "Breastfeeding and the Use of Human Milk," *Pediatrics* 129, no. 3 (March 2012): e827–841, https://1ref.us/21f (accessed June 7, 2022).

210 J Rosenbauer, P Herzig, G Giani, "Early Infant Feeding and Risk of Type 1 Diabetes Mellitus," *Diabetes/Metabolism Research and Reviews* 24, no. 3 (Mar–Apr 2008): 211–222, https://1ref.us/21v (accessed June 7, 2022).

211 U Das, "Breastfeeding Prevents Type 2 Diabetes Mellitus: But, How and Why?" *The American Journal of Clinical Nutrition* 85, no. 5 (May 2007): 1436–1437, https://1ref.us/21w (accessed June 7, 2022).

212 L Horwood, D Fergusson, "Breastfeeding and Later Cognitive and Academic Outcomes," *Pediatrics* 101, no. 1 (January 1998): E9, https://1ref.us/21x (accessed June 7, 2022).

213 "Breastfeeding and the Use of Human Milk."

214 M Kramer et al., "Effects of Prolonged and Exclusive Breastfeeding on Child Behavior and Maternal Adjustment: Evidence from a Large, Randomized Trial," *Pediatrics* 121, no. 3 (March 2008): e435–440, https://1ref.us/21y (accessed June 7, 2022).

215 B Vohr, "Persistent Beneficial Effects of Breast Milk Ingested In the Neonatal Intensive Care Unit," *Pediatrics* 120, no. 4 (October 2007): e953–959, https://1ref.us/21z (accessed June 7, 2022).

216 A Lucas, R Morley, T Cole, "Randomised Trial of Early Diet In Preterm Babies and Later Intelligence Quotient," *British Journal of Medicine* 317 (November 1998): 1481–1487, https://1ref.us/220 (accessed June 7, 2022).

217 E Isaacs et al., "Impact of Breast Milk on Intelligence Quotient, Brain Size, and White Matter Development," *Pediatric Research* 67, no. 4 (April 2010): 357–362, https://1ref.

Breast milk helps pass meconium

Babies are born with a sticky tar-like substance called meconium in their intestines. Colostrum, or early milk, is uniquely designed to help move this substance through the infant's body.

Breast milk is more digestible than formula

Babies can digest human milk more easily than the milk of other animals, probably because human milk contains an enzyme that aids in this process. Breast milk forms softer curds in the infant's stomach than cow's milk (the basis for most formulas) and is more quickly assimilated into the body system. While it contains less protein than does cow's milk, virtually all the protein in breast milk is available to the baby. By contrast, about half the protein in cow's milk passes through the baby's body as a waste product. Similarly, iron and zinc are absorbed better by breastfed babies.

Pre-term milk is specially designed for premature infants

Milk produced by women who deliver prematurely differs from that produced after a full-term pregnancy. Specifically, during the first month after parturition, preterm milk maintains a composition similar to that of colostrum.[218]

Formula-fed babies have a higher risk of developing certain childhood lymphomas[219]

Breastfeeding decreases chances of juvenile rheumatoid arthritis[220]

Formula-fed babies are more at risk for obesity in later life[221]

---

us/221 (accessed June 7, 2022).

218 M Underwood, "Human Milk for the Premature Infant," *Pediatric Clinics of North America* 60, no. 1 (February 2013): 189–207, https://1ref.us/222 (accessed June 7, 2022).

219 Z Gao et al., "Protective Effect of Breastfeeding Against Childhood Leukemia In Zhejiang Province, P.R. China: A Retrospective Case-control Study," *Libyan Journal of Medicine* 13, no. 1 (2018): https://1ref.us/223 (accessed June 7, 2022).

220 E Kindgren, M Fredrikson, J Ludvigsson, "Early Feeding and Risk of Juvenile Idiopathic Arthritis: A Case Control Study In a Prospective Birth Cohort," *Pediatric Rheumatological Online Journal* (2017): 46, https://1ref.us/224 (accessed June 7, 2022).

221 "Breastfeeding vs. Formula Feeding," KidsHealth, https://1ref.us/225 (accessed June 7, 2022).

Breast milk always has the right proportions of fat, carbohydrates, and protein

Formula companies are constantly adjusting these proportions looking for the best composition. The reality is that a mother's milk composition changes from feeding to feeding depending on the needs of her child.

Breastfed babies are healthier overall[222]

Cow's milk is designed for baby cows

Human milk contains completely different proportions of protein, fat, carbohydrates. Cow's milk is designed to help put on weight quickly, grow amazingly fast, and develop only as much brain power as a cow needs. The hormones in cow's milk are geared toward cows, not humans. The fact that human beings can even drink the milk of another species is sort of amazing when you stop to think about it.

Human milk is designed for baby humans
Baby cows would not do very well on it. It is designed to build brains and to foster gradual physical growth.

Natural pain relief for baby[223]
Breast milk actually contains chemicals that suppress pain (endorphins). Aside from this, the comfort a baby derives from being held close and suckling is remarkable. The pain and trauma of many a bruise or scrape has been soothed away almost instantly by a few moments of nursing. If you choose to have your child vaccinated, it is a good idea to nurse immediately after he/she receives a vaccination. This soothes the hurt, as well as enhancing the vaccine's effectiveness.

Perfect food for sick baby[224]
When a formula-fed baby gets a gastrointestinal ailment, they are usually put on an artificial electrolyte solution because formula is too hard for them to digest. Breast milk, however, is easily digested, and soothing to the intestines, so there is no need for artificial and expensive electrolyte

---

222 "Breastfeeding vs. Formula Feeding."
223 "Mother's Milk As a Natural Painkiller," WebMD, https://1ref.us/226 (accessed June 7, 2022).
224 H Becker, "Viral Photo Shows How Breastmilk Changes for Baby's Needs," *Parents*, January 21, 2020, https://1ref.us/227 (accessed June 7, 2022).

solutions. If a baby gets a respiratory illness, formula may cause even more mucus. In contrast, breast milk contains antibodies to these ailments, as well as being highly digestible and not contributing to excess mucous formation.

Facilitates proper dental and jaw development[225]
Suckling at the breast is good for a baby's tooth and jaw development. Babies at the breast have to use as much as sixty times more energy to get food than do those drinking from a bottle. As [the baby's jaw] muscles are strenuously exercised in suckling, their constant pulling encourages the growth of well-formed jaws and straight, healthy teeth.

Among breastfed infants, the longer the duration of nursing, the lower the incidents of malocclusion.[226]

Better cognitive development
In a study of 771 low birth weight infants, babies whose mothers chose to provide breast milk had an eight-point advantage in mean Bayley's mental developmental index over infants of mothers choosing not to do so.[227]

Decreased risk of baby developing urinary tract infections[228]

225 X Wang, L Ge, "Influence of Feeding Patterns on the Development of Teeth, Dentition and Jaw In Children," *Journal of Peking University* 47, no. 1 (February 2015): 191–195, https://1ref.us/228 (accessed June 7, 2022).

226 M Boronat-Catalá et al., "Association Between Duration of Breastfeeding and Malocclusions In Primary and Mixed Dentition: A Systematic Review and Meta-analysis," *International Journal of Scientific Reports* 7 (2017): 5048, https://1ref.us/229 (accessed June 7, 2022).

227 R Morley, T Cole, R Powell, A Lucas, "Mother's Choice to Provide Breast Milk and Developmental Outcome," *Archives of Disease In Childhood* 63, no. 11 (November 1988): 1382–1385, https://1ref.us/22a (accessed June 7, 2022).

228 R Chamova et al., "Protective Effect of Breast Milk on Urinary Tract Infection In Children Aged 0–3 Years," *Journal of IMAB* 24, no. 1 (Jan–Mar 2018): 1918–1922, https://1ref.us/22b (accessed June 7, 2022).

ADDITIONAL READING

Chapter 1

Bowman, Chris. "Plant saved millions by breaking rules." *Fresno Bee,* December 12, 2004.

———. "Reports of nonstop pollution from cheese factory spur action." *Fresno Bee,* March 24, 2005.

Chen, Robert. *Milk, The Deadly Poison.* Englewood, New Jersey: Argus Publishing, Inc., 1997.

Keith Schneider. "Lines Drawn in a War Over a Milk Hormone." *New York Times*, March 9, 1994, p. A12.

———. "F.D.A. Warns the Dairy Industry Not to Label Milk Hormone-Free." *New York Times*, February 8, 1994, p. A1.

Statement of Michael Hansen, Ph.D., Research Associate Consumer Policy Institute, Consumers Union on FDA's Safety assessment of Recombinant Bovine Growth Hormone, December 15, 1998.

Kathleen Day, "Hormone Hubbub Hinders Program," Washington Post, March 15, 1994, pp. D1, D5.

Michael K. Hansen, *Biotechnology and Milk; Benefit Or Threat? An Analysis of Issues Related to BGH/BST Use in the Dairy Industry* (Mount Vernon, N.Y.: Consumers Union/Consumer Policy Institute, 1990), p. 3.

Michael Hansen, Ph.D., Jean M. Halloran, Edward Groth III, Ph.D., Lisa Y. Lefferts, "Potential Public Health Impacts Of The Use Of Recombinant Bovine Somatotropin In Dairy Production, Prepared for a Scientific Review by the Joint Expert Committee on Food Additives," September, 1997.

Lippman, M., "IGF-I is critically involved in the aberrant growth of human breast cancer cells." J. Natl. Inst. Health Res., 1991, 3.

Lee, A.V., "Estrogen regulation of IGF-I in breast cancer cells would support the hypothesis that IGF-I has a regulatory function in breast cancer." Mol-Cell- Endocrinol., March, 1999(2).

Chen, J.C., "IGF-I is a potent growth factor for cellular proliferation in the human breast carcinoma cell line." J-Cell-Physiol., January 1994, 158(1).

Figueroa, J.A., "Insulin-like growth factors are key factors for breast cancer growth.", J-Cell-Physiol., November 1993, 157(2).

Musgrove, E.A., "IGF-I plays a major role in human breast cancer cell growth." Eur-J-Cancer, 29A (16), 1993.

"IGF-I has been identified as a key factor in breast cancer." The Lancet, vol. 351. May 9, 1998.

Lippman, M., "IGF-1 accelerates the growth of breast cancer cells", Science, Vol. 259, January 29, 1993.

Chapter 2

VIROLOGY June3, 2009 (PMID:19494004).

Veterinary Research 25(1994):521.

Johnson J., "Molecular biology and pathogenesis of the human T-cell leukaemia/lymphotropic virus Type-1 (HTLV-1)". Int J Exp Pathol. 2001 Jun;82(3):135-47.

Cancer Research 34(1974):2745

"AIDS Research and Human Retroviruses" 19(2003):1105. Science 213(1981):1014.

Journal of Virology Methods 104(2002): 33.

American Journal of Epidemiology 112 (1980):80.

British Journal of Cancer 61(1990):454.

Hulse, Virgil, *Mad Cows and Milk Gate* (Phoenix, Oregon: Marble Mountain Publishing, 1996).

Gonda M., "Bovine immunodeficiency virus. AIDS". 1992 Aug;6(8): 759-76.

Whetstone, C.A., "Examination of whether persistently indeterminate human immunodeficiency virus type 1 Western immunoblot reactions are due to serological reactivity with bovine immunodeficiency-like virus". J ClinMicrobiol. 1992 Apr;30(4):764-70.

Jacobs, R.M., "Detection of multiple retroviral infections in cattle and cross-reactivity of bovine immunodeficiency-like virus and human immunodeficiency virus type 1 proteins using bovine and human sera in a western blot assay". Can J Vet Res. 1992 Oct;56(4):353-9.

Ferrer, J.F., "Milk of dairy cows frequently contains a leukemogenic virus". Science. 1981 Aug. 28;213(4511):1014-6.

Kim, S. G., Kim, E. H., Lafferty, C. J., & Dubovi, E. (2005). Coxiella burnetii in bulk tank milk samples, United States. *Emerging infectious diseases*, 11(4), 619–621. https://doi.org/10.3201/eid1104.041036.

Chapter 3

Eisnitz, Gail, *Slaughterhouse* (Prometheus Books: New York 1997).

Chapter 4

Agricultural Statistics from The National Agricultural Statistics Service, https://1ref.us/21p.

USDA Food Safety and Inspection Service, https://1ref.us/21q.

Animal Disposition and Reporting System, https://1ref.us/21r.

Chapter 5

James, Robert E., "Feeding management to reduce the Environmental Impact of Dairy Farms," Department of Dairy Science, and Beverly Cox, Virginia Cooperative Extension. Published in the University of Florida IFAS, 45th Dairy Conference Production proceedings.

EPA Region 9 Pacific Southwest, https://1ref.us/21s.

Weida, W., "A CITIZEN'S GUIDE To The Regional Economic and Environmental Effects of Large Concentrated Dairy Operations," Dept. of Economics, The Colorado College, Colorado Springs, CO; November 19, 2000.

Sell, R., Knutson L., "Quality of Ground Water in Private Wells in the Lower Yakima Valley 2001-2002," Valley Institute for research and Education, December 2002.

Innes, R. "The Economics of Livestock Waste and Regulation." *American Journal of Agricultural Economics* 82 (February 2000): 97-117.

Nelson, J., "South Dakota's dairy industry continues to grow," Dairy Star, 10/25/2010.

Watanabe, N., "Environmental Occurrence of Antibiotics in Dairy Farming," Pare No. 5-12, 2008. Joint Meeting of The Geological Society of America, Soil Science Society of America, American Society of Agronomy, Crop Science Society of America, Gulf Coast Association of Geological Societies with the Gulf Coast Section of SEPM.

Burgos, J.M., Ellington, B.A., Varela, M.F., "Presence of Multi-Resistant Enteric Bacteria in Dairy Farm Topsoil," Journal of Dairy Science, vol. 88, Issue 4, April 2005, 1391-1398.

Robert E. James, Department of Dairy Science, and Beverly Cox, Virginia Cooperative Extension. "Feeding management to reduce the Environmental Impact of Dairy Farms," Published in the University of Florida IFAS, 45th Dairy Conference Production proceedings.

Capper JL, Cady RA, Bauman DE. The environmental impact of dairy production: 1944 compared with 2007. J Anim Sci. 2009 Jun;87(6):2160-7. doi: 10.2527/jas.2009-1781. Epub 2009 Mar 13. PMID: 19286817.

Arnold, Stephen, PhD, "Dairy Herds and Rural Communities in Southern New Mexico", July-August 1999, Environmental Health, p.11.

Wen-yuan Huang and Sara D. Short, "The Economic Impacts of EPA's CAFO Rule on Dairy Farms in Cornbelt, upper-Midwest, and Northeast regions," Paper prepared for presentation at 2002 annual AAEA meeting, Long Beach, California, July 28-31.

J. Burkholder, R. Libra, P. Weyer, S. Heathcote, D. Kolpin, P. S. Thorne, and M. Wichman. 2007. "Impacts of waste from concentrated animal feeding operations on water quality". Environ. Health Persp. 115(2):308-312.

J. L, Capper, E. Castañeda-Gutiérrez, R. A. Cady, and D. E. Bauman. 2008. "The environmental impact of recombinant bovine somatotropin (rbST) use in dairy production". PNAS 105:9668-9673.

Chapter 6

Akers, A., *A Vegetarian Sourcebook* (G.P. Putnam's Sons: New York, New York, 1983), p. 30.

"Amino Acids in Nutrition and Growth," *Journal of Biological Chemistry*, 17:325, 1914.

Sanchez, A., Scharffenberg, J, Register, U.: "Nutritive Value of Selected Proteins and Protein combinations," *American Journal of Clinical Nutrition*, vol.13 #4, October 1963, p. 247.

Marieb, E.N., *Human Anatomy and Physiology* (Benjamin/Cummings Publishing Company Inc.: Redwood City, CA., 1989), pp. 487–8.

Marsh, A., Sanchez, T., Chaffee, F., Mayor, G., Mickelsen, O., "Bone Mineral Mass in Adult Lacto-ovo Vegetarians," *American Journal Of Clinical Nutrition*, March 1983, pp. 453–456.

Marsh, A., et. al., *American Journal of Clinical Nutrition*, 1988:48 pp. 837–41.

Heaney, R.P., "Protein intake and bone health: the influence of belief systems on the conduct of nutritional science," *American Journal of Clinical Nutrition* 73:5, 2001.

Sellmeyer, D.E., "A high ratio of animal to vegetable protein increases the rate of bone loss and the risk of fracture in postmenopausal women," *American Journal of Clinical Nutrition* 73:118, 2001.

Lock, J., Board, R., "Persistence of Contamination of Hen's Egg Albumin in vitro with Salmonella Serotypes," *Journal of the American Medical Association*, December 23, 1992, p. 3428.

Consumer Reports, Feb. 1992, pp. 103-104.

Health News and Review, Spring 1992.

"Transmission of Salmonella by Intact Chicken Eggs," *American Family Physician*, January 1992, P. 355.

"Raw eggs are no yolk," *Medical Update*, August 1991, p. 3.

Journal of the American Medical Association, June 24, 1992, p. 3263.

American Journal of Clinical Nutrition, 1988:48 pp. 754-61.

Chapter 7

European Journal of Clinical Nutrition, 1994 (48:305–325).

Davies, "Antibodies and Myocardial Infarction," The Lancet, ii: 205–207, 1980.

Ornish, Dean, *Dr. Dean Ornish's Program for reversing Heart Disease* (New York: Ballantine Books, 1990), p. 76.

Mepham, T.B., "Safety of Milk from Cows Treated with Bovine Somatotropin," Lancet. July 16, 1994. 344(8916):197–8.

Juskevich, J.C., "Bovine Growth Hormone: Human Food Safety Evaluation," Science, Aug 24, 1990. 249(4971):875–84.

Holmes, M.D., "Dietary Correlates of Plasma Insulin-like Growth Factor I and Insulin-like Growth Factor Binding Protein 3 Concentrations," Cancer Epidemiol Biomarkers Prev., Sept. 11, 2002. (9):852–61.

Cadogan, J., "Milk Intake and Bone Mineral Acquisition in Adolescent Girls: Randomized, Controlled Intervention Trial," BMJ, 1997; 315:1255–1260.

Heaney, R., "Dietary Changes Favorably Affect Bone Remodeling in Older Adults," J Am Diet Assoc, 1999, 99:1228–33.

Janowski, T., "Mammary Secretion of Oestrogens in the Cow," Domest Anim Endocrinol. July 23, 2002, (1-2):125–37.

British Medical Journal, October 7, 2000, 321:847–848.

Yu, H., "Role of the Insulin-like Growth Factor Family in Cancer Development and Progression," J Natl Cancer Inst., Sept. 20, 2000, 92(18):1472-89.

Buehring, G.C., "Evidence of Bovine Leukemia Virus in Human Mammary Epithelial Cells," Vol: 3 Abs: V-1001 1997, Pg:27A.

Journal of AIDS Research and Human Retroviruses (December 27, 2003).

Lancet. April 24, 2004: 363(9418):1346–53.

Journal of the American Medical Association (JAMA 2003): 289: pp. 1421-4.

Cancer Epidemiology, Biomarkers Prevention (June18, 2009): (6):1881–7.

Judith C. Juskevich and C. Greg Guyer. SCIENCE, vol. 249.

August 24, 1990. "IGF-I is critically involved in the aberrant growth of human breast cancer cells."

Lippman, M.J., Natl. Inst. Health Res., 1991, p. 3.

Figueroa, J.A., J-Cell-Physiol., November, 1993, 157(2).

Chen, J.C., J-Cell-Physiol., January, 1994, 158(1).

Lippman, M. Science, Vol. 259, January 29, 1993

Heaney, Robert P., Journal of the American Dietetic Association, vol. 99, no. 10. (October 1999).

Morimoto, L.M., Newcomb, P.A., White, E, Bigler, J, Potter, J.D.: Variation in plasma insulin-like growth factor-1 and insulin-like growth factor binding protein-3: personal and lifestyle factors (United States). Cancer Causes Control (2005): 16:917–927.

Holmes, M.D., Pollak, M.N., Hankinson, S.E., Lifestyle correlates of plasma insulin-like growth factor I and insulin-like growth factor binding protein 3 concentrations. Cancer Epidemiol Biomarkers Prev (2002): 11:862–867.

American Journal of Epidemiology, (March 1, 2004; Volume 159, Issue 5): pp. 454466 Science 1986;233(4763).

Abelow, B., Cross-cultural association between dietary animal protein and hip fracture: a hypothesis. Calcific Tissue Int 50:14–8, (1992).

Frassetto, L.A., Worldwide incidence of hip fracture in elderly women: relation to consumption of animal and vegetable foods. J Gerontol A Biol Sci Med Sci. (2000 Oct): 55(10):M585–92.

"Increasing one's protein intake by 100% may cause calcium loss to double." Journal of Nutrition, (1981): 111 (3).

Maurer, M., Neutralization of Western diet inhibits bone resorption independently of K intake and reduces cortisol secretion in humans. Am J Physiol Renal Physiol. (2003 Jan): 284(1):F32–40.

Remer, T., Influence of diet on acid-base balance. Semin Dial. 2000; Jul–Aug; 13(4):221-6.

Frassetto, L., Diet, evolution and aging—the pathophysiologic effects of the post agricultural inversion of the potassium-to-sodium and base-to-chloride ratios in the human diet. Eur J Nutr. (2001 Oct): 40(5):200–13.

Remer, T., Potential renal acid load of foods and its influence on urine pH. J Am Diet Assoc. (1995 Jul), 95(7):791–7.

American Journal of Clinical Nutrition (1979): 32(4).

Recker, R.R., The effect of milk supplements on calcium metabolism, bone metabolism and calcium balance. Am J Clin Nutr. (1985 Feb): 41(2):254–63.

December 28, 2008 volume of Food Nutrition Research (Cho K, Cederholm T. 2008;52. doi: 10.3402/fnr.v52i0.1654).

A 1994 study published in the American Journal of Clinical Nutrition (Remer, T., Am J Clin Nutr 1994; 59:1356–61).

American Journal of Clinical Nutrition, (1995): 61 (4).

New England Journal of Medicine (July 30, 1992): page 302, Karhalainen, et al.

Cavallo, et al. LANCET, October 1996 348; 926-928.

LANCET, vol. 348, Dec 14, 1996.

Pediatrics, 1992; 89; 1105–1109.

European Journal of Clinical Nutrition (2005 Mar): 59 (3):393–8.

American Journal of Epidemiology (2005 Feb): 161(3):219–27.

LANCET, (1992): 339, 905–909.

Iacono, G., Intolerance of cow's milk and chronic constipation in children. N Engl J Med. (1998 Oct 15): 339(16):1100–4.

Journal of Pediatrics, (1990): 116.

Journal of Pediatric Surgery, (1999 Oct): 34:10.

Lancet (2004): 363:5–6, 39–40.

Ryan, C.A., Nickels, M.K., Hargrett-Bean, N.T., Potter, M.E., Endo, T., Mayer, L., et al. Massive outbreak of antimicrobial-resistant salmonellosis traced to pasteurized milk. JAMA (1987): 258:3269–74.

Dalton, C.B., Austin, C.C., Sobel, J., Hayes, P.S., Bibb, W.F., Graves, L.M., et al. An outbreak of gastroenteritis and fever due to *Listeria monocytogenes* in milk. N Engl J Med (1997): 336:100–5.

Ackers, M.L., Schoenfeld, S., Markman, J., Smith, M.G., Nicholson, M.A., DeWitt, W., et al. An outbreak of *Yersinia enterocolitica* O:8 infections associated with pasteurized milk. J Infect Dis (2000): 181:1834–7.

Black, R.E., Jackson, R.J., Tsai, T., Medvesky, M., Shayegani, M., Feeley, J., et al. Epidemic *Yersinia enterocolitica* infection due to contaminated chocolate milk. N Engl J Med (1978): 298:76–9.

Centers for Disease Control and Prevention. *Salmonella* gastroenteritis associated with milk—Arizona. MMWR Morb Mortal Wkly Rep (1979): 28:117–20.

Tacket, C.O., Narain, J.P., Sattin, R., Lofgren, J.P., Konigsberg, C. Jr, Rendtorff, R.C., et al. A multistate outbreak of infections caused by *Yersinia enterocolitica* transmitted by pasteurized milk. JAMA (1984): 251:483–6.

Fleming, D.W., Cochi, S.L., MacDonald, K.L., Brondum, J., Hayes, P.S., Plikaytis, B.D., et al. Pasteurized milk as a vehicle of infection in an outbreak of listeriosis. N Engl J Med (1985): 312:404–7.

Centers for Disease Control and Prevention. Salmonellosis from inadequately pasteurized milk—Kentucky. MMWR Morb Mortal Wkly Rep (1984): 33:505–6.

Birkhead, G., Vogt, R.L., Heun, E., Evelti, C.M., Patton, C.M. A multiple-strain outbreak of Campylobacter enteritis due to consumption of inadequately pasteurized milk. J Infect Dis (1988): 157:1095–7.

Journal of Dairy Science (1992): 75(9):2339.

Guggenmos, et al., Journal of Immunology (2004 Jan 1): 172(1):661–668 (The Lancet 1974; 2:1061).

Neuroepidemiology 1992; 11:304?12.

Maurin, M., Raoult, D.Q., fever. Clin Microbiol Rev. 1999; 12:518–53.

McQuiston, J.H., Childs, J.E., Q fever in humans and animals in the United States. Vector Borne Zoonotic Dis. 2002; 2:179–91.

Willems, H., Thiele, D., Frolich-Ritter, R., Krauss, H., Detection of Coxiella burnetii in cow's milk using the polymerase chain reaction (PCR).

Zentralbl Veterinarmed, B. 1994; 41:580–7.

Kim, S. G., Kim, E. H., Lafferty, C. J., & Dubovi, E. (2005). Coxiella burnetii in bulk tank milk samples, United States. *Emerging infectious diseases*, 11(4), 619–621. https://doi.org/10.3201/eid1104.041036

Chapter 8

Schernhammer, E.S., Hankinson, S.E., Hunter, D.J., Blouin, M.J., Pollak, M.N.: Polymorphic variation at the -202 locus in IGFBP3: Influence on serum levels of insulin-like growth factors, interaction with plasma retinol and vitamin D and breast cancer risk. Int J Cancer 2003, 107:60–64.

Setiawan, V.W., Cheng, I., Stram, D.O., Penney, K.L., Le Marchand, L., Altshuler, D., Kolonel, L.N., Hirschhorn, J., Henderson, B.E., Freedman, M.L.: IGF-I genetic variation and breast cancer: the multiethnic cohort. Cancer Epidemiol Biomarkers Prev 2006, 15:172–174.

American Journal of Clinical Nutrition, Vol. 86, No. 6, (December 2007): 1722–1729,

"ICF and colo-rectal cancer," British Journal of Cancer (2001) 85, 1695–1699. doi:10.1054/bjoc.2001.2172

The International Journal of Cancer (Ganmaa, et al. 98:262–267.

Chaoyang, Li, Ph.D., Wei Xin, M.D., and professor of pathology, Man-Sun, Sy, Ph.D, September issue of the Journal of Clinical Investigation.

"Dietary Fatty Acids and Pancreatic Cancer in the NIH-AARP Diet and Health Study," J Natl Cancer Inst (2009) 0: djp233v1-969 June 26, 2009. 101: 1001-1010.

International Journal of Cancer (Jun 10 ,2004);110; 2: 271–7) 1999.

The American Journal of Epidemiology, (Volume 150) Lancet (1989).

IGF Carcinogenesis, doi:10.1093/carcin/bgp257.

Chan, June M., et al. "Insulin-like growth factor-1 (IGF-1) and IGF binding protein-3 as predictors of advanced-stage prostate cancer," Journal of the National Cancer Institute, Vol. 94, (July 17, 2002,) pp. 1099–1106.

Chan, June M., "Insulin-like growth factor-1 (IGF-1) and IGF binding protein-3 as predictors of advanced-stage prostate cancer," Journal of the National Cancer Institute, Vol. 94, (December 18, 2002), pp. 1893-94.

British Journal of Cancer (April 1, 2008).

European Journal of Urology, Volume 3, (March 2004) pp 271–279).

Giovannucci, E., Adv Exp Med Biol 1999; 472:29–42.

Bosetti, C., Eur J Cancer Prev 2000, Apr; 9 (2):119–23.

Snowdon, D.A., Am J Epidemiol 1984, Aug; 120 (2): 244–50.

Trends Mol Med. 2005 Feb; 11(2): 52–55.

Djavan, B., Waldert, M,, Seitz, C., Marberger, M.: "Insulin-like growth factors and prostate cancer." Grimberg, A., Cohen, P., "Role of insulin-like growth factors and their binding proteins in growth control and carcinogenesis," J Cell Physiol 2000, 183:1-9 World J Urol 2001, 19:225–233.

Wolk, A., Mantzoros, C.S., Andersson, S.O., Bergstrom, R., Signorello, L.B., Lagiou, P., Adami, H.O., Trichopoulos, D., "Insulin-like growth factor 1 and prostate cancer risk: a population-based, case-control study." J Natl Cancer Inst (1998), 90:911–915.

Lawrence Erlbaum Associates, Inc., Antonella Dewell, Gerdi Weidner, Michael D. Sumner, R. James Barnard, Ruth O. Marlin, Jennifer J. Daubenmier, Christine Chi, Peter R. Carroll, and Dean Ornish "Relationship of Dietary Protein and Soy Isoflavones to Serum IGF-1 and IGF Binding Proteins in the Prostate Cancer Lifestyle Trial,". NUTRITION AND CANCER 2007, 58(1), 35–42.

Chapter 9

Owen, F., Poulter, M. Collinge, J. Leach, M., Shah, T., Lofthouse, R., Chen, Y.F., Crow, T.J., Harding, A.E., Hardy, J., et al. Division of Psychiatry, Clinical Research Centre, Harrow, Middlesex, United Kingdom. Exp Neurol 112 (1991): 240–2.

Massoud, F., Devi, G., Stern, Y., Lawton, J.E., Goldman, Y., Liu, S., Chin, S., Mayeux, R. "A Clinicopathological Comparison of Community-Based and Clinic-Based Cohorts of Patients With Dementia," Arch Neurol, November 1, 1999; 56(11): 1368–1373.

Teixeira, F., et al. "Clinico-Pathological Correlation in Dementias," Journal of Psychiatry and Neuroscience 20 (1995): 276–282.

Kelleher, Colm. *Brain Trust*. New York, NY: Pocket Books a division of Simon & Schuster, 2004.

McKhann, Guy, et al. "Clinical Diagnosis of Alzheimer's Disease." Neurology 34 (1984): 939.

DeArmond, S.J., Curr Opin Neurol 6: 872–81 (1993).

Glabe, C., "Intracellular mechanisms of amyloid accumulation and pathogenesis in Alzheimer's disease." J Mol Neuroscience 2001 Oct; 17(2):137–145.

Brown, Paul. "Central Nervous System Amyloidoses," Neurology 39 (1989):1103–1104.

Pratico, D., Clark, C.M., Liun, F., Rokach, J., Lee, V.Y., Trojanowski, J.Q., "Increase of brain oxidative stress in mild cognitive impairment: a possible predictor of Alzheimer disease," Arch Neurology 2002 Jun; 59(6): 1475.

Rhodes, Richard. *Deadly Feasts*. New York: Simon & Schuster, 1997.

Giem, P., Beeson, W.L., Fraser, G.E., "The incidence of dementia and intake of animal products: preliminary findings from the Adventist Health Study," Neuroepidemiology 1993; 12(1):28–36.

David A. Snowdon, PhD; Lydia H. Greiner, BSN; James A Mortimer, PhD; Kathryn P. Riley, PhD; Philip A. Greiner, DNsc; William R., Clinical Expression of Alzheimer Disease, The Nun Study; JAMA 1997; 277: 813817.

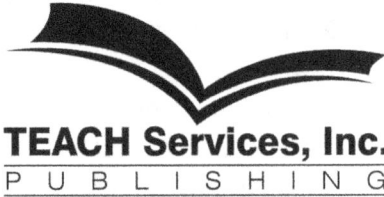

www.ingramcontent.com/pod-product-compliance
Lightning Source LLC
Chambersburg PA
CBHW070918270326
41927CB00011B/2620